Eating Your Way to a Healthy Lifestyle

BY KICKING THE DEVIL OUT!

Janet A. Cooksey

This book or parts thereof may not be reproduced in any form, stored in a retrieval system, or transmitted in any form by any means – electronic, mechanical, photocopy, recording, or otherwise – without prior written permission of the publisher, except as provided by United States of America copyright law.

All scripture quotes are from the King James Version (KJV) unless otherwise noted.

Design Director: Janet A. Cooksey

ISBN: 978-197383572X
ISBN-13: 978-1973835721

DEDICATION

This book is dedicated to my beautiful and handsome son, Antoine. You were born for such a time as this. Without you always standing by me and cheering me on, I wouldn't be where I am. You are my Great Encourager. You lift me up and inspire me to continue being a healthier and better me, even training me in how to do certain exercises and stretches. Yes, I have a personal trainer who pushes me to no end, not only in physical fitness but in life. Thanks, Son, with much love for you. Thanks for being the best son a mother could hope for.

This book is also dedicated to the memory of my dear parents, Charlie and Pearl Cooksey who chose to bring me into this world, nurture, and love me. I missed that they will not get a chance to this birthed in the natural but I know spiritually they are looking over the balcony of heaven cheering me on. Thanks for being a part of my cheering section in the cloud of witnesses.

ACKNOWLEDGMENTS

I acknowledge my Lord and Savior Jesus Christ. I thank Him for helping me to birth this book and giving the grace and revelation to share with others. Without Him, there is nothing. The word says, I can do all things through Christ who strengthens me.

I acknowledge, my Sister, my Friend Serena Eason. She has read and given many comments, insight and wisdom during the writing of this book. She listens to my complaints, my grumblings but she encouraged me to the end to complete this book. Even say get that one done you have another one. Keep going. Thank you Serena, for sticking it out with me to help me push this out.

To my sister Norma, I always hear her voice you can do this and I believe in you. Thank you dear sister for always holding me up, when I needed it the most.

ENDORSEMENTS

I love the unique approach that Janet took with this book. It takes into account that we are a triune man -- addressing our spirit with prayers and declarations, our soul with testimonies and a journal section, and our body with lifestyle tips and recipes. Janet is an anointed woman of God, whom I have the honor and privilege of serving alongside of in ministry. I know for a fact, that the section on how to eat and what to eat came straight from the Throne Room. I pray this book blesses you as it did me. - Serena Eason, Aneres Ministries COH - IAM Ministries

I have been blessed and experienced personal healing and deliverance by reading this book during the process of editing. I have known Janet a long time and know her to be a true woman of God, pure in heart and motive. Her heart is to encourage and help everyone she comes into contact with. Her motive for writing this book is to see more people healed and delivered from sickness and general mediocrity, due to not feeling great, than she could reach on a personal basis. Do yourself a favor and read this book but not only read it. Follow what it says. You will be blessed. - Vickie Marlin, Editor

CONTENTS

1

INTRODUCTION

This book is written for those who struggle with eating properly, emotional eating, eating disorders, food addictions, yo-yo diets, excessive supplements, obesity and properly maintaining a healthy lifestyle. The everyday struggle of losing and releasing the excess weight and keeping it off. I honor you for wanting a healthy lifestyle and maintining proper weight. To desire and want to take control of your life. It hasn't been easy up till this point, so let's just say keep climbing up the mountainside until you reach the top. Determine within yourself that this is the time and make a choice right now that you will achieve your goal and fulfill your destiny. That you will be healthy and living in your best body yet and will achieve it. Honor and respect your body to attain it.

Now, you will have to do something! You will have to get active! You will have to eat properly! Will it be hard? Yes, but it's worth it. This maybe the hardest decision you have to make to live and thrive again. This book is not about just losing the excess weight, it is about getting rid of the weight that is killing your soul. What do I mean by that is unearthing the emotional pain, deep hurt, the scars from your past that keep festering because they are not dealt with. They have been swept under the rug. Now, it is time to clean house, to do a "spiritual detox." To clean your soul (mind, will and emotions), heart, gateways and body.

Truth be told, I thought I was pretty healthy until my life drastically changed in 2012. I was always busy doing something. Whether it was pursuing business endeavors or ministry opportunities, I was basically always on the go. I was never one to eat on a planned schedule. Sometimes I forgot to eat at all during the day.

On one occasion, I was at a meeting on a job site. It wasn't supposed to last long. During those days I always wore high heels. You know, I had be cute and all.

We had our meeting in a computer mainframe operations center where we stood up the entire time. After awhile, I started feeling faint so I grabbed a nearby chair. It was too late. I hit the floor and was out for a few minutes. Yes, I fainted.

Of course, I was at the age where people tend to feel invincible. I thought that attitude was working for me but was actually causing harm to my body. I scared myself and everyone else. Even though I laughed it off to ease the embarrassment, they wanted to haul me off in an ambulance. Of course I refused. The manager in charge asked me several questions.

The first one was, "Are you pregnant?"

I said "No."

The second one was, "When was the last time you've eaten anything?"

I couldn't remember the last meal or even most recent snack, so they shoved an apple at me and I ate that.

After that incident, everyone in my office paid attention to whether I had eaten and they reminded me when the cafe was getting ready to close, to go get lunch. You talk about accountability. I had more than I wanted. It was great, though, to know people really cared enough to watch over me. They sometimes even brought lunch for me when they noticed I had gotten busy and skipped it again.

Even though I'd had a scare, my pattern remained to be more concerned about weight gain than good health. In my mind, I had to be in a perfect body. That's where I needed to renew my mind from what the world said I needed to be and looked like. To be honest, most of us have been brainwashed to believe that we should be a size this or that to be beautiful or healthy. Really we were looking for acceptance and approval in the world but not within our hearts.

As a youth and young adult, I was always the skinny one and I loved it. I would never gain weight, no matter how much I ate. When I would visit home, my mother and aunt would get behind us younger women, if we were going out together, and they would say things like, "Look. She's gained weight. She's even getting some hips!"

I guess, in their minds, I was too thin. They were glad to see me filling out. Nowadays, people are not so kind about whether you are thin or full figured. If you are thin, they say you must be on crack. If you are full figured, they think you just need to stop eating so much, you know, turn your plate over.

One must be careful what they are saying because you maybe cursing and projecting illwill to another person unknowinlgy and unintentionally. This was an area I had to deal with that I didn't recognize that I had wounds in my soul tat occurred at a young age but the fruit of that manifested later on in life. I also made inner vows and unjust judgments against my mother and sister, as well as others about their weight. I repented and asked for forgiveness for these sins against them. I confronted my sister aand she forgave. But in the case with my mother who is now in heaven,

I went before the Lord and repented and ask forgiveness.

So, getting back to the fainting scare and the subsequent kind encouragement from coworkers, I decided I wanted to be healthy and live. I really needed to take control of my life before it was too late.

Getting back to what happened in 2012 - I was diagnosed with breast cancer in the left breast, in the lymph node under my armpit. That was one of the scariest moments in my life. You talk about a wake up call. The alarm was blaring very, very loudly.

I had taken my yearly mammogram a year earlier with no reported evidence of any lumps or illness. So I went along my way, happy-go-lucky for the most part. But I stayed stressed out due to workaholism, performance anxiety and perfectionism. I felt I had to prove to the world and myself that I was "good enough." This all goes back to undealt heart issues that I had swept under the table, the sting of rejection kept rising up.

What I didn't know then was that something was physically eating at my body while negative emotions were eating at my soul and I was spiritually immature in a lot of areas. This was definitely not what the Word of God had promised me as an abundant life.

Almost a year after the 2011 annual mammogram, during a monthly breast self-examine, I found a lump in that area. After seeking medical advice, I had a lumpectomy done. I must say I was ignorant then about that kind of thing and didn't do due diligence. While waiting on the results, I received a phone call and was advised to get another opinion. I was recommended to a specialist in this area and immediately received an appointment based on my history. I was rushed through the process of getting a MRI, which the first surgeon didn't mention that was necessary. After the initial consultation, I was shown the film from the year before and the current one side by side. The surgeon was greatly displeased because she immediately saw the lump in the film from the previous year. So I had the lump there for a year. After my decision to proceed with biopsies on both breasts it was determined to have the lump removed and radiation treatments and medications. After that, I was given recommendations to change my diet and eat right. I will not go into all the details about that but now I am cancer free.

If you're wondering whether I truly changed my eating habits and lifestyle. I did at first, but didn't stick with it long enough. I started noticing a pattern. When I was worried about someone or something - most times my son, as he was living overseas or the many doctor visits and radiation or determining whether to take chemotherapy - I would lapse into emotional eating and it caused me to gain weight. After the treatments, I started taking meds and that caused more weight gain. I felt my biggest enemy was getting on that scale on every office visit. I was alive and well, so I still had purpose, strength and the will to turn this around.

So, imagine every time you stepped on a scale see a sledge hammer smashing that scale to smithereens which represents the weight is coming off. Whether it is ounces or pounds keep moving forward, remember to keep looking up to the mountain peak. Another way is to post a picture of yourself that you see every day, visualize yourself already there. Do this every day, maybe several times a day. Another way is to purchase a dress or suit the size you are desiring to be and keep it in your eye gate every day. You may have an item in your closet right now that you are desiring to get in again, a great pair of jeans or slacks pull them out so that you can see them everyday. Plan a day in the future, a date with your new self with the item you planned to wear and treat yourself to a special day of achieving your goal. Do this often - "Celebrate" your accomplishment. Take it one day at a time and track all of your changes in the daily journal.

Understand the devil's tactics, he will try one way then another and continue to keep from fulfilling your destiny. In your mind you will hear or your body will crave - carbs, sugary foods, etc. Have to get a handle on that. That's why it is important to recognize where you have abused your body so you can take authority and take back what the devil stole.

Finally, enough was enough and I recognized, with God's help, that I needed to be healed from the inside out. I had to discover my weaknesses and what triggered me to eat or crave food when I wasn't hungry. I had to know what was driving me to eat. What prompts you in the middle of the night to wake up from a deep and head straight to the kitchen "to eat". But what do I grab usually chips, cookies or something sweet. Where is this unhealthy urge coming from? Is it a habit? or What is the source behind it?

Reviewing my life, I realized I was constantly doing what I grew up doing, without much thought about it. The foods we ate back then were the same foods I found myself consuming. I cooked them the same way, too. I found out that I really didn't know how to eat properly. I realized most people follow the examples we saw growing up, without question as to why or if it was the best way. Mostly, our family culture and traditions prevailed. I believe as you continue to read and get activated you will see those things being broken off of you.

Secondly, I needed deliverance from the trauma, wounds and pains of my past. I could no longer dwell on the past. I wanted and needed to let those things go. I had to drop off the excess baggage. I sought out resources that could help me but knew I had to help myself first.

In that time, I faced the fact that I needed guidance and had to let go of pride and arrogance. I got rid of the attitude that I could do it by myself. I had to stop lying to myself and others that I was alright and own the fact that I was dealing with depression, self-hatred, oppression, stress, anxiety and fear. It had become an everyday battle. Sometimes, just to get out of bed each day was just that - a battle. So, when someone asks me today how are you my response is "Better than I was yesterday". No more lying saying I'm fine or I'm good.

Sharing about it wasn't always easy though. Someone would say, "You're a Christian, right?"

Of course, I answered each time, "Yes."

It was painful to learn that not everyone knew how to deal with others in love, even though they meant well. I learned to keep my guard up, as I would immediately get turned off by Christian brothers' and sisters' comments like, "You need to pray more, fast more." I needed Christian Shadowing Boxing at this time because you wanted to hit someone but you could hit the air or even hit a boxing bag.

Some even asked, "Where is your faith?"

Those conversations added guilt and condemnation to a heart that was already hurting. That's what made me feel worse than anything, the finger pointing. Isaiah 58:8-9 says, *"Then shall thy light break forth as the morning, and thine health shall spring forth speedily: and thy righteousness shall go before thee; the glory of the LORD shall be thy reward. ⁹ Then shalt thou call, and the LORD shall answer; thou shalt cry, and he shall say, Here I am. If thou take away from the midst of thee the yoke, the putting forth of the finger, and speaking vanity..."*

I know I am speaking for others, as well, when I talk about these kinds of responses causing pain, hurting instead of helping.

On that note, I want to set the record straight. If I could write a letter, from my heart and on behalf of others, to all who have been hurt the same way, here's what it would say. In fact, I am saying it. "I apologize for every unkind word or wayward look that came your way. If the way I looked at you made you feel less than and ugly, I'm sorry. I'm even sorry for where I have ever overlooked you and called you names. Forgive me for my ignorance and lack of maturity, but most of all, forgive me for not caring enough to reach out a loving hand. Forgive me for not having compassion for you. Forgive me for the slightest thing that made you feel uncomfortable. Forgive me for my finger pointing. No, I'm not responsible for all that happened to you, but I'm sorry it happened. Forgive me, Yours Truly, Janet."

I hope that helps and lets you know you're not alone. With all the original hurts I harbored, plus the pain piled on by judgmental statements and attitudes of those I turned to for help and release, more than ever, I needed help and the Lord led me to focus on the area of eating.

I came upon a teaching about the Courts of Heaven. Intrigued at this new and exciting idea, I begin searching this out for myself. I want to say here it was new to me but as timeless as God. I realized soon that the Bible, God's Word, is a legal document, filled with courtroom language, all designed to help and protect us.

In this first part of my journey, I read many books and watched several informative videos on the subject. In the process, I gained some divine connections;

people God led me to, who could help me in the area I was seeking understanding in.

In watching one of the videos about abuse to our bodies that cause infirmity, I was prompted to ask the question, "In what ways have I abused my body?"

This video showed me the process of the courts of heaven and how I could allow my body to take me to court with its complaints against the way I had treated it.

In the natural, we know what "being taken to court" means. If there is a cause against you, someone may take you to court.

After seeing this video, I allowed my body to take me to court. I wanted to know what I had done to allow sickness, disease, physical ailments, etc., to come upon my body. I was overwhelmingly surprised at the charges or accusations my body had against me. I know this sounds a little "out there," but your body talks to you. If something is not functioning properly in your body, discomforts such as pain, fever, headaches, sleeplessness and other ailments will let you know something is off and needs to be dealt with. Might as well get to the root, which is internal I call soul wounds, rather than patching it with any assortment of bandages of other forms of abuse (alcohol, drugs, etc) which cover it but don't truly deal with the cause.

With the knowledge I had gained, I sought the Lord and prepared the case about the abuse my body had suffered. One of the areas of mistreatment was poor diet; another was lack of exercise.

I sought the counsel of the Lord asking for wisdom on eating properly. What I found out was I didn't really know how to eat properly. I was still doing the things I learned growing up simply because that's what was done. We ate what we could afford. We ate the traditional meals our families grew up on through many generations. That was our comfort zone and even if something new was introduced, it took some time for the family to try it.

Now, someone might ask, "Does God really care about what you eat?"

"YES," with all capitals!

During one session with the Lord in His boardroom, where I was in a heavenly visitation, there was set in front of Him some bread, wine and a donut!

I said, "I want the bread and the wine but I want that donut, too!"

He knows me well and knew I would say that. In that time in His Presence, He gave me instructions on how to eat properly and laid out His plan on how to do so.

A lot He shared with me was about foods I didn't eat at the time but He said I would begin to enjoy them after my body detoxed from the old way of eating and started experiencing the new habits.

Also, I must say this. It is time I kicked the devil, the bully, out of my life. It is time to kick some devil butt. He had been killing me slowly and put blinders on me, without me knowing his devices. If he can't get me one way, he will try another. He suckered Eve in the garden and I was getting suckered in the garden, as well!

So, I say to you the reader are you ready to kick the devil out of your life. Open the door and kick the bully out. No more being deceived! We want tolerate deception any longer.

That being said, this book is designed to help you on your journcy of Eating to a Healthier Lifestyle! In it, you will find helpful tips and simple, light recipes.

I didn't count calories. One thing I did was drink more water and another was to add more alkaline foods to my diet. But there's more about that in the pages that follow. Remember, this is a lifestyle change, not a diet.

Areas that is covered in this book is:
- Maintaining the pH (potential for hydrogn) balance of the body
- Doing a spiritual detox
- Why have an alkaline diet
- Tips to increase the alkaline in your body
- What foods to eat
- How to check your pH balance
- Sample meal plan to get you started
- Daily Journal to track your progress daily
- Recipes to start with or add tour meal plans
- Prayer of Activation for Supernatural Weight Loss
- Daily Declarations to encourage you every day and speak over yourself for 7 days

It's time to get started!

2
DAILY DECLARATIONS

As I stated in the introduction, my trigger for eating was that I needed inner healing. There were emotional wounds in my soul that caused me to grab the snacks, the sugary sweets and yes, donuts, eating late at night even when I wasn't hungry.

I have a story about the donuts, as referred to in the introduction, but most may not believe it. On this occasion, a group of us wanted to seek the counsel of the Lord. We were led to a boardroom where we sat down with Jesus Christ to consult with him. We all had some questions but since we were in his presence, I asked the question about supernatural weight loss. He laughed but he also stated it didn't come on that way. I knew then I must do my part and he would help me to do what I needed to.

Another note on the doughnuts, I love sweets and yes I love doughnuts. A few days prior to the session I ate a package of the small cake doughnuts which I knew I shouldn't have, but I did. Why, because I just wanted it or there was a trigger. So, I believe this is why that was placed before while in the presence of the Lord, what am I going to choose going forward. I had to start making wise decisions on what to eat, do not yield to temptation. I must have self control in every decision and choice of what I decide to eat. Eat what is good.

If I didn't intentionally pursue getting the emotional wounds healed in my soul, and even if I lost the weight I wanted to lose, I knew it could come back if I didn't change the patterns or habits in my life. So, my road to a healthy lifestyle started inside. Getting rid of past hurts, disappointments, trauma, bitterness, anger, and unforgiveness is where it all started. Repentance for sins, transgressions and iniquities of myself and my forefathers all the way back to the beginning of time.

Anything that would cause me to continue in old, unhealthy patterns had to go. I had to face a hard truth that I didn't love myself because I didn't believe I was worthy. I devalued myself and always tried to prove my value to others. However, no matter what I did on the outside, it wasn't making a change on the inside.

I have tried diet plans, exercise, fasting, and supplements, which worked for a while until I started eating regular again. Because I was focused on the outside and not targeting the triggers of why I was eating emotionally, under stress and worry and constant weight gain. Sometimes, it seemed as if I looked at a cookie or slice of cake I would gain 5 pounds. That's not the reality I want to continue to live. I need to be healthy, strong and vibrant, alive and well in my spirit, soul and body. So, it is best to work on all three areas of your body for total health and wholeness. By now you know I am a believer in Jesus Christ. Yes, I have fallen short of the glory of God, who hasn't especially in taking care of my temple.

So, life happens. What do you do? What I planned didn't go as planned. What I expected to happen wasn't happening the way I expected. Unmet expectations bring disappointment. I had to change my mind and the ways I lived my life. I had be intentional about my life and be transformed from the inside out. I couldn't say it is what it is, which is something I don't like saying or hearing anyone say it. What we speak out of our mouths either creates or destroys. If we don't speak change then it will not change. I started speaking to my body, mind, soul and spirit to line with the word of God and I had to raise my expectations.

One thing I had to do was pronounce over myself daily declarations of who I am, my identity in Christ. After I took the case about abusing my body to court to be judged. I also started pronouncing declarations over my body.

I know you are asking, "What do you mean - to court?" I mean courts of heaven. Yes, I touched on this earlier, but I feel the need to put it in terms that one would understand, my body had accusations against me, charges against me in the heavenly courts that I didn't know about. So, how did I find out that, there were accusations against me or that I needed to do this. What I have found out is that as Christians in some respect have thought that everything just happens for you, you don't have to do anything. Even though salvation was paid for us, we had to take a step of faith and confess our sins and accept Jesus Christ as our Lord and savior. We know every promise in the word of God belongs to us; the finished work of the cross belongs to us. However, all has to be appropriated in our lives. Some of the promises there are conditions that need to be met. No, it just doesn't happen in the natural. This is not magic and God is not a magician. His will is done, not ours. The word of God says, the accuser goes about like a roaring lion looking for someone to devour and the enemy seeks to detour us in fulfilling our destiny. Revelation 12:10 *And I heard a loud voice saying in heaven, Now is come salvation, and strength, and the kingdom of our God, and the power of his Christ: for the accuser of our brethren is cast down, which accused them before our God day and night.*

Basically, if you have wronged someone or thing there can be charges drawn up against you in a court of law. I was accused of: poor diet, not drinking enough water, not resting properly, too much sleep at times, being sedentary, diet plans, not eating God's way, unforgiveness, self-hatred, self-rejection, worry, stress, depression, offense, bingeing, fear, pride, arrogance, familiar spirits, witchcraft, idolatry, bitterness, believing the lies of the enemy and trauma to name a few. I had to appear before the just judge and listen to these accusations against me and my bloodline. Knowing that I had a clear advantage because I have the blood of Jesus covering me. I said I was guilty of all charges and repented for them and any others brought forth. No, this is not a crash course on the courts of heaven but I hope it reveals that to you that your body may have a case against you. There are over 100+ accusations that have been accumulated that the body can charge you with. Yes, let me clarify one more thing, it is your body that is the temple of the Holy Spirit, but the accuser brings up the charges. You have to be aware that the accuser goes around like a roaring lion seeking whom he may devour. He has been devouring us in the way we eat and how we take care of our temples. We have been in a slumber and stupor not realizing that this is a wile of the devil. For most Christians, the devil can't accuse us of murder, but he can find the little foxes, and how we have not taken care of our temples, etc. We have not been attuned to this tactic of the enemy, we just didn't care, it's too hard or we just didn't know what to do.

In my research and ministry time, I have found that most people need healing and deliverance from the following: freemasonry (number one), witchcraft (number two) and deaf and dumb spirit (number three). I am not saying that you are demonically possessed, but maybe influenced or attacked in some way.

Second, in this process, you have to be brutally honest and transparent to get the results you want. Get rid of shame, guilt and embarrassment right now. Open the door, keep them out. For me, I needed deeper inner healing and I sought out for help. Initially, I went to healing room for prayer and other ministry associates to pray for me on many occasions. Watch many ministers on supernatural weight loss, healing and deliverance. I studied and read many books on self-deliverance, which I did. But I needed more. I had a SOZO (saved, healed, delivered) session which is a unique inner healing and deliverance ministry to get to the root of things that were hindering my personal connection with the Father, Son and Holy Spirit. But I also had to address some deep seeded issues that I didn't want to confront. I had to face why I reacted the way I did when I got frustrated or off kilter.

So, now about the body. I had to start eating healthy, alkaline foods, drinking more water and adding exercise. That's why I included the tips section in this book to help you jumpstart your program.

Finally, I decided to engage God gateways of the spirit, soul and body. Each of the gateways needed to be cleansed from any defilement that I had allowed to come in, even from birth. For example, my ear gateway may have gotten defiled has an infant due to certain types of music playing on the television unnoticed by my parents, that subtleness of the enemy again. This caused wounds to my soul as an infant. Another example, my eye gateway got defiled through television from watching shows like Bewitched, I Dream of Jeannie, vampire movies, and scary movies. Guess what at the time we thought that was cute and fun, but it opened the door to witchcraft, nightmares, night terrors and black magic, which also caused wounds to my soul. Do you see a pattern here? Everything that you are exposed too may have an effect on your life and your gateways. Therefore, you must protect them at all times. I also believe this also affects you losing weight and having an abundant life. See Engaging God Gateways(1) for more information.

Finally, one must recognize that this is a total makeover for life. Change the way you have been taught to lose weight. Change the way you have been taught to eat and what an how to eat. Doing time management on when you are to eat (putting yourself on schedule to eat). Paying close attention to what foods you are eating and how it works with your body.

Preparing healthy dishes that fit and work for you.

So, where am I right now? Working my program so that I can live a life to the fullest vibrantly, strong, and healthy. Have I achieved my goal totally? Not yet, because this is a lifestyle change, not a diet plan or a quick fix! I will be working this for the rest of my life.

I hope that this has really encouraged you to continue with the reading of this book and start the program. I have included this prayer of activation of supernatural weight loss and healthy eating. This is used to activate your faith and your activity to do something. This is not a magic trick. This prayer is a prayer of repentance as well and following declarations you speak over your body. I recommend that you can pray the declarations daily. Before doing this prayer, spend some time in praise and worship.

Prayer for Activation of Supernatural Weight Loss and Healthy Eating

I decree and declare that as you pray this prayer with expectancy and fervency the anointing for supernatural weight loss be activated in you now. I pray that the Holy Spirit helps you and strengthen you in your inner man. I decree that angels are dispatched to you to have charge over you.

Father, in the name of Jesus I repent and renounce

for the way I have abused my body, in any way, shape or form, including excessive exercise, not getting the proper rest, denial, speaking negativity over my body, not loving my body the way God made me, having addictions and addictive behavior. I repent and renounce of coming into agreement, any involvement and allowing any of the following strongholds and all of its manifestations in the midst of me and my family line at any time: anger, fear, abandonment, shame, lying, financial lack, addictions, sensuality, depression, grief, mental instability, pride and procrastination. I repent and renounce any eating disorders, gluttony, guilt, shame and embarrassment. I repent for believing the lies of the enemy, negative words spoken over and about me, idolizing my body, excessive supplemental use and other means.

In Jesus Name, I ask that my ministering angels to pull out all of the enemy's weapons of destruction: daggers, darts, knives, swords, spears, javelins, machetes, axes, tomahawks, bullets, projectiles, voodoo pins and hatchets in my back, sides, head, hands, feet, any part of my body that have been thrown knowingly, unknowingly, intentional or unintentional, of hatred, anger, rage, betrayal, false accusations, character assassination, offense, envy, jealousy, lying, slander, unjust judgments, strife, division, murder, pain, revenge, spite, death wishes against me, etc., throughout my lifetime, even when I

was in my mother's womb and even back to Adam! Expose any that may have lodged in any part of my body: liver, lungs, heart, womb, groin, etc.
Lord, I ask you to pour your healing Balm of Gilead over the wounds Lord, nullify the poison, the sting, and nullify the venom in Jesus' name.

I break every word curse, witchcraft curse, national curse, generational curse, hex, spell, vex, hoodoo, juju, voodoo, jinx, joke, incantation off of me from the crown of my head to the soles of my feet. I also break every soul ties to every witch, warlock, sorcerer, occultist, satanist, religious manipulator that maybe connected via social media and websites (facebook, youtube, vimeo, periscope, etc.) and any other channel unknown to me but known to God.

I also break off, pull off every silver cord, band, rope, chain, wire any all instruments and/or devices used by the enemy to bound me or caused death and destruction from any evil and demonic sources, entities, secret societies.

I break off any defilement, contamination or pollutant off of me. I speak that all of my gateways are cleansed in Jesus' name.

I render all of the above impotent, null and void. They are cancelled and I command every record with my name on it to be removed and burned by the fire of God.

I repent and renounce any form of offense, of where I got offended and where I caused someone else to get offended. I release all offense, bitterness, resentment, malice and hatred now. I apply the blood of Jesus over my soul right now, into every wound in my soul from the abuse to my body where I caused the wounds or anyone else did, any wounds from sickness and disease, sin, unrighteousness, anything not of love and all forms of trauma, especially emotional trauma that has been locked in any part of my body. I command all emotional traumas to be unlocked in every part of my body to be unlocked. Any PTSD be unlocked and released from my body, soul and spirit. I release all of that as an act of my will. I now receive the goodness of God, forgiveness, peace, healing, deliverance and restoration in Jesus name.

I repent and renounce of not loving myself. I repent of binge eating. I repent of ever believing and saying that God must hate me. I repent and renounce self-loathing, foreboding and self-pity. Forgive me Lord for giving up and giving in to the enemy's trap of trying to destroy and kill me before my time. I repent and renounce all forms of rejection, rejection from my mother's womb, not being wanted by my parents, rejection from siblings and family members, rejection of man and even rejecting myself, before others could. I repent and renounce illegitimacy off of my bloodline and me. I repent and renounce any and all word curses off of me from my parents wanting a different sex child causing a curse to come upon me. I repent and renounce any failed attempts of abortion, abortion as a means of birth control, idle talk of abortion, murder and shedding of innocent blood. I repent and renounce of fear, anxiety and stress that came upon me from my mother's womb, umbilical cord and the birth canal. I repent and renounce suicide, self-hatred, self-rejection, self-mutilation and premature death off of me, right now.

I release everyone and even myself that have caused me hurt, pain, abuse, grief, trauma and any of the above. I forgive them and myself. I release them into total forgiveness right now. I ask you Lord to bless them and have mercy on those who are deceased. Thank you Jesus!

I apply the blood of Jesus over my life right now, from the crown of my head to the soles of my feet.

I break off depression, oppression, suppression, anxiety, fear, menopause, mid-life crisis and all word curses that have ever been spoken over my life, even back, to when I was in my mother's womb. I speak to my DNA, RNA, and mitochondria to be cleansed and restored by the blood of the lamb, and aligned with the divine word of God.

I command all forms of sickness and disease in the digestive system be healed, made whole and healthy. I speak health and healing to all of my body. I speak strength to my body and command all functions of my body to be restored and functioning properly in Jesus' name.

I speak over myself supernatural weight loss. I speak that my body will come into agreement and alignment with this prayer of activation and declarations now. I speak and I hug my body right now, I love you body, I love you and hug you right now.

Now, I decree for the release of the breaker anointing over you to break every barrier and hindrance that have held you in bondage. I break every stronghold, band and cord and I release myself now into the new me, healthier me, toner me, and stronger me. I renounce and break off all demonic spirits, demonic entanglements now, in Jesus' name. Father, I decree that everything that Jesus has carried is lifted from me now and Jesus rise up with healing in His wings over my life and flood me with your glory and light.

I ask for wisdom Father on how to proceed and to take steps necessary for a healthy lifestyle. I ask you

Lord to supernaturally cleanse my palette and desire to choose the wrong foods. Help me to make the right choices with food choices, exercise and spiritual health. Help me to change any poor health habits. I ask that Holy Spirit energize me each and every day to exercise and strengthen my body. I ask for fresh vigor, vitality and clarity of mind. I desire to put you first in my life, Lord help me to do that.

And now declare - I decree and declare I will do what I need to do on a daily basis to change my lifestyle. I will be intentional. I will be conscious of what I am doing each day. I will be bold and courageous. I can do this! I will do this. I must be intentional. Lord with your grace and your help I can do this and achieve a healthier me. I will live and not die. I will live and not die!

Daily Declarations to Speak Over Your Body

Pronounce these daily declarations over your body. Ask for the grace of God every day before doing these declarations.

Day 1 – Scripture References: 2 Corinthians 12:9 And he said unto me, My grace is sufficient for thee: for my strength is made perfect in weakness. Most gladly therefore will I rather glory in my infirmities, that the power of Christ may rest upon me. Philippians 4:13 I can do all things through Christ which strengtheneth me. Proverbs 18:21 - Death and life are in the power of the tongue: and they that love it shall eat the fruit thereof.

1. I ask and receive grace, wisdom, revelation and strength today in the name of Jesus.

2. I speak right now over my body, I love you and I hug you right now.

3. I am sorry where I have abused you but today I want to do all that I can to honor, respect and protect you. To bring health and wholeness to you. I pray for your cooperation and that you engage in this with me and not fight against me. We are in agreement with one another.

4. I decree that I have a sound body and sound mind.

5. I decree I have the mind of Christ because I am a child of God.

6. I speak life and health to my soul, body and spirit.

7. I decree that my body is not feeble.

8. I declare and decree over my body to function properly in every way...

9. Every organ in my body to function properly.

10. Every muscle, tendon, ligament return to

proper strength and length.

11. I command my skeletal system to come into alignment with the head, proper height be restored, legs grow out to the same length, arms grow to the same length.

12. I command any and all curvature in my spine to come out and my spine to straighten now in Jesus' name.

13. I command my thyroid gland to function properly.

14. I command my thyroid gland to be rebooted and recharged.

15. I command my glandular system to be rebooted and recharged.

16. I command my parathyroid gland to function properly.

17. I command my thymus gland to function properly

18. I command my hypothalamus to function properly.

19. I command my pituitary gland to function properly.

20. I command any abnormal swelling in the pituitary gland to shrink now.

21. I command my brain to send the proper communication signals to my body, soul and

spirit.

22. I command every negative thought to be uprooted and plucked out my mind, will and emotions.

Day 2 – Scripture References: Luke 1:37 For with God nothing shall be impossible. Luke 18:27 And he said, The things which are impossible with men are possible with God. Mark 11:24 Therefore I say unto you, What things soever ye desire, when ye pray, believe that ye receive [them], and ye shall have [them].

23. I command all emotional trauma, abuse of every type, psychologically, physiologically, biologically, economically, mentally, financially, relationally, socially and any other channel to be unlocked and plucked out of my body, soul and spirit from the time I was being conceived in my mother's womb to the present and all the way back to Adam and a thousand generations forward.

24. I command all damage to be reversed, to be brought back into alignment with the perfect will of God.

25. I command the hormones in the pituitary gland to be normal, in harmony and balanced. To be corrected now.

26. I command any abnormal growths, masses,

cysts and tumors to shriveled up and die right now. I curse that spirit causing these growths to leave me now and be cursed at the root of conception. Every one of the growths I released the atomic fire of God to them now.

27. I command that the proper Leptin hormone is at the proper level and signals my body is full when needed.

28. My body is not insulin resistant; it properly regulates the insulin throughout my body.

29. I command my metabolism to be restored to proper level and function in my body.

30. I command my appetite control center to function properly.

31. I command my hormonal, chemical and magnetic frequencies to be balanced and harmony in my body.

32. I command the frequency of the brain to return to normal range of 72-90 MHz.

33. I command the frequency of my body to return to normal range of 62-78 MHz.

34. I command the frequency of the body from the neck up to return to normal range of 72-78 MHz.

35. I command the frequency of the body from the neck down to return to normal range of 60-68

MHz.

36. I command the frequency of the thyroid to return to normal range of 62-68 MHz.

37. I command the frequency of the parathyroid glands to return to normal range of 62-68 MHz.

38. I command the frequency of the thymus gland to return to normal range of 65-68 MHz.

39. I command the frequency of the stomach to return to normal range of 58-65 MHz.

40. I command the frequency of the colon to return to normal range of 58-63 MHz.

41. I command the frequency of the spleen to return to normal range of 60-80 MHz.

Day 3 – Scripture References: Proverbs 3:6 In all thy ways acknowledge him, and he shall direct thy paths. Proverbs 3:8 It shall be health to thy navel, and marrow to thy bones. Proverbs 4:22 For they are life unto those that find them, and health to all their flesh.

42. I command the frequency of the heart to return to normal range of 67-70 MHz.

43. I command the frequency of the lungs to return to normal range of 58-65 MHz.

44. I command the frequency of the pancreas to return to normal range of 60-80 MHz.

45. I command the frequency of the liver to return

to normal range of 55-60 MHz.

46. I command any sugar or fructose that I have consumed in my body that it will not block the burning of fat in my body.

47. I command the excess fat cells to shrink in my body.

48. I command my muscles to be firm and toned.

49. I command my pancreas and endocrine system to process insulin properly and regulate blood sugar levels properly.

50. I command any toxins stored in the adipose tissue/fat tissue to be released properly from the body.

51. I command my liver to function properly to filter out toxins and waste from my blood.

52. I command my kidneys to function properly and the bile duct to function properly.

53. I command my body to have a good and healthy good bile flow.

54. I command all constipation, PMS, toxicity and disease to leave my body now in Jesus' name.

55. I command my small intestine, large intestine, colon, and rectum to function properly.

56. I command the spirit of death to come out of any part of my body.

57. I command the spirit of affliction to leave my body.

58. I speak life to every part of my body.

Day 4 – Scripture References: Isaiah 58:8 Then shall thy light break forth as the morning, and thine health shall spring forth speedily: and thy righteousness shall go before thee; the glory of the LORD shall be thy reward. Proverbs 16:24 Pleasant words are as honeycomb, sweet to the soul, and health to the bones. Jeremiah 33:6 Behold, I will bring it health and cure, and I will cure them, and will reveal unto them the abundance of peace and truth.

59. I come against liver stress and command the liver to be healed, strengthened and total health to be restored.

60. I command every manifestation/symptom of liver and gallbladder problems to cease and desist.

61. I command the pH balance to be normal, balanced and harmony in my body.

62. I command my blood sugar level to be normal.

63. I command my blood pressure to be normal.

64. I command my vascular system to be healthy and whole.

65. I command all traumatic water to be eliminated

from the body.

66. I command all water locked in the lymphatic system to be unlocked and eliminated from my body.

67. I command that my lung capacity increase for the proper oxygen supply and flow.

68. I break every word curse of edema and lymphedema off of me.

69. I command any excessive, overgrowth of Candida and yeast to be destroyed, dissolved and discarded from my body.

70. I command all residue, symptoms and any damage caused by the overgrowth of Candida and yeast to cease and desist now. All gastrointestinal disturbances to stop: gas, bloating, irritable bowel syndrome, colitis, psoriasis, and skin disorders and crohns disease.

71. I command memory loss, depression, problems concentrating, memory fog and severe fatigue to cease and go from me now in Jesus' name.

72. I command the production and balance of good bacteria to be restored and maintained in my body.

73. I command all parasites to be eliminated from my body.

74. I command all bad and overgrown bacteria and

fungi in my body to cease and desist production in excess, and all overgrown bacteria to be discarded and eliminated from my body inside and out. In all layers of skin and all organs, any part of my body now, in Jesus' name.

75. All toxins and free radicals be eliminated from my body.

Day 5 – Scripture References: 3 John 1:2 Beloved, I wish above all things that thou mayest prosper and be in health, even as thy soul prospereth. Malachi 4:2 But unto you that fear my name shall the Sun of righteousness arise with healing in his wings; and ye shall go forth, and grow up as calves of the stall. Matthew 4:23 And Jesus went about all Galilee, teaching in their synagogues, and preaching the gospel of the kingdom, and healing all manner of sickness and all manner of disease among the people.

76. I command that the proper level of glutathione is produced in the body to get rid of lead, arsenic and mercury out of the body.

77. I release and apply the blood of the Lamb to nullify the toxins and the poisons in my body.

78. I command my immune system, my defense system of my body to be strengthen, fortified, healed and restored, where it has been

compromised may it be restored, healthy and whole to ward off all microorganisms: germs, viruses, bad bacteria, fungi and infections that invade the body.

79. I command the spirit causing joint aches and stiffness to come out of my body.

80. My immune system is rejuvenated, revitalized, energized, invigorated and refreshed to secure and protect my body.

81. All water retention excess water is eliminated.

82. I command all bloating to cease.

83. I will lose the excess weight.

84. I will lose the weight from the result of medications that I have taken. I break off every symptom and reverse that in Jesus' name.

85. I will not overeat any longer; my leptin hormone is level and activated in my body.

86. My muscles are toned and firmed.

87. My skin return to normal elasticity and all stretch marks is removed.

88. I command all sickness, affliction, disease, infection, germs, bacteria, virus that tries to come upon me die now, by the blood of Jesus.

89. No plague, no evil entity nor storm shall come near my dwelling in the name of Jesus.

90. I command every aspect of my life, body, soul and spirit to come into alignment with the word of God. By his stripes I am healed.

91. Lord, let your kingdom come, let your will be done in my life, health, body, soul, spirit, finances, relationships as it is in heaven.

92. I have a healthy heart and lungs.

93. I can breathe normally because my lungs are healed, healthy and strong.

Day 6 – Scripture References: Psalms 23:3 He restoreth my soul: he leadeth me in the paths of righteousness for his name's sake. Psalm 51:12 Restore unto me the joy of thy salvation; and uphold me with thy free spirit. 2 Samuel 22:33 God is me strength and power; and he maketh my way perfect.

94. I will lose weight supernaturally even in my sleep.

95. I will get the proper sleep for my body.

96. I will drink proper amounts of water

97. I will do the proper exercise.

98. I will do all of this by the grace of God.

99. I speak now over my soul now that all dross, chaff, wood, hay, stubble, every briar and thorn are burned by the fire of God.

100. I ask that the fire of God to purify me

and my soul from every wound that has caused me to be bondage of any kind, but specifically weight gain or obesity.

101.   I pray that every device that the enemy has used against me to caused death, destruction and loss be destroyed and leave me now and go to the feet of Jesus for judgment.

102.   I ask for a download of the Father's heart and love, mercy, compassion, grace, his goodness to flood me right now. Every empty place to be filled by the Holy Spirit.

103.   I speak to every element of the periodic table that is part of the natural composition of my physical body to return to normal levels, corrected and balanced.

104.   Any elements of the periodic table that is not a normal part of the natural composition of my physical body to be eliminated from my body.

105.   I speak that my genetic makeup, chromosomes and all genes be touched and restored by the hand of God. May the blood of Jesus cleanse them, in Jesus' name.

106.   I command the frequency, resonance and sound of each strand of the DNA in each chromosome to be corrected.

107.   I command any additions or mutations to

the chromosomes or genes that the enemy has made be repaired and corrected.

108.   Anything that has been extracted or removed by the enemy I call it back now into the proper position and placement.

109.   I cancel out everything that has been injected into my body knowingly or unknowingly through food and drink, pesticides, fertilizers and any other chemical that modifies plant and animals genetics, Genetically Modified Organism (GMO), Hormone Replacement Therapy (HRT), blood transfusions, soul ties, animals, vaccines, transplants, reptilian, medications, prescriptions, chemotherapy, and other substances that has caused harm in any form or fashion to be eliminated, deleted from my body now. All residue be eliminated. I pray all of that to be reversed into health, wholeness and soundness.

110.   I command that every trigger, trauma, grief, unforgiveness, pain, hurt, deep hurt, repressed memories, defense and coping mechanism all be removed at the root of conception.

Day 7 – Scripture References: 2 Samuel 22:40 For thou hast girded me with strength to battle; them that rose up against me hast thou subdued under me. 1 Chronicles 16:11 Seek the LORD and his strength, seek his face continually. Isaiah 53:5 But he was wounded for our transgressions, he was bruised for our iniquities; the chastisement of our peace was upon him; and with his stripes we are healed.

111. I lay the axe to the root now in Jesus' name.

112. I ask that God's eraser, erases all of this now and forever and that I walk in divine health and wholeness.

113. I call myself and all of the fragments of my soul from the ungodly depths, ungodly stars, out of captivity now in Jesus' name.

114. I command every gate that should be opened, be opened. Every gate that should be closed, be closed.

115. I command every door that should be opened, be opened. Every door that should be closed, be closed.

116. I pray that all of this is accomplished by the finished work of Jesus Christ on the cross.

117. I also apply the blood of Jesus over this work.

118. Thank You Lord for all that you are doing in my life, body, soul and spirit.

119. Thank you that You want me whole,

healed and having an abundant life.

120.   Thank you that You have delivered me from the hands of my enemies.

121.   Thank you that you set a table before me in the presence of my enemies.

122.   Thank you for the renewed strength, hope, love, joy, and peace.

123.   Thank you that you love me with an everlasting love. Even when I turned away from you, when I didn't love myself. You still love me.

124.   Thank you for never leaving me nor forsaking me.

125.   Thank you for delivering me from myself, where I caused myself harm, hurt and abuse.

126.   Thank you for bringing me out of darkness into your marvelous light.

127.   Thank you for flooding me with your glory and light like you did the woman with the issue of blood.

128.   Thank you for your grace and mercy that you bestowed upon me; even when I was like Saul of Tarsus, I persecuted you. I blamed you and pointed my finger at you.

129.   Thank for the precious blood of Jesus

and the finished work of the cross. Because I receive all and appropriate all of this in and through my life today.

130.   I am redeemed from the curse of the law.

131.   I also appropriate and receive the blessings from Deuteronomy 28.

132.   By the stripes of Jesus I am healed. Amen.

Salvation Prayer

Scripture References: *Titus 2:11 For the grace of God that bringeth salvation hath appeared to all men, Jonah 2:9 But I will sacrifice unto thee with the voice of thanksgiving; I will pay that that I have vowed. Salvation is of the LORD. Romans 10:10 For with the heart man believeth unto righteousness; and with the mouth confession is made unto salvation.*

For those who want to accept Jesus Christ as your Lord and Savior, as your Master Builder, Restorer and Creator of your life and all that concerns you right now, just say, Jesus I accept you as my Lord and Savior, come into my heart and be enthroned over my life from this day forward. I recognize you as my Creator and I now agree with the finished work of the cross. I now appropriate all of that to my life, body, soul and spirit. Because I choose Life today. I choose the Tree of Life. Amen.

3
TIPS FOR HEALTHY LIFESTYLE

This chapter contains 24 tips on helping you reached your goal of a healthy lifestyle.

Tip 1.	**Water Intake**

Upon arising in the morning, drink 2 glasses of water. This helps the organs in the body. You can also drink a full glass of warm water when you first get out of bed. This will help the digestive system to eliminate waste.

Before each meal, drink a full glass of water. This will help you to not overeat. You will get full faster.

Drink a glass of water before your bath to help lower blood pressure.

Drink a glass of water before bed to help prevent heart attacks, strokes and leg cramps.

Tip 2:	**Drink Warm Water**

Tip 2: Again, drink a full glass of warm water first thing in the morning, even before brushing your teeth. It cleanses your digestive system. This is very good for those who have sluggish digestive tracts.

Tip 3:	**Sugar Cravings**

If you fill like you are hungry and are reaching for sugary snacks/food, drink a full glass of water. Note: Sugar makes you hungry

Tip 4:	**Drink Apple Cider Vinegar (ACV)**

Note: Recommend - Certified Bragg Organic Raw Apple Cider Vinegar - organic, unfiltered, with the Mother. Can be taken 3 Times a day

Mixture #1:

1 teaspoon of Bragg Apple Cider Vinegar

8 ounces of mountain spring water

Optional - 1-2 teaspoons of 100 % Organic Honey, Maple Syrup

Optional - Add a pinch of cayenne pepper (Cayenne Pepper helps to lower blood pressure).

Mixture #2:

Mix 2 parts apple juice and 2 teaspoons ACV

Mixture #3:

Mix 2 parts grapefruit, orange or pineapple juice and 1 part ACV

A. Drink in the morning after you eat.

B. Drink again before supper, and eat immediately.

Tip 5:	**Increase the alkaline in your diet**

Be careful with the oranges, don't over do the oranges.

Tip 6:	**Apple Cider Skin Toner**

You may have skin breakouts because your body will start detoxification.

You can use Apple Cider Skin Toner. Depending on your skin type I would blend 1 part ACV and 1 part water. Use cotton ball to apply to clean skin. You may also use full strength if the skin breakouts are that severe. I use the toner at night before bed.

Tip 7:	**Lemon/Lime Water**

Drinking lemon/lime water increases the enzymes to help detoxify your liver

Use Organic Lemons/Limes and mix with 8 ounces of mountain spring water and drink slowly. Remember, if you get the urge to eat something sugary reach first for a glass of lemon water instead.

**Note: Sugar makes you hungry.

Tip 8:	**Eating Bread**

You may eat bread but limit to 3 times a week. That is the maximum

Tip 9:	**Red Meats**

Eat red meats in moderation. It takes more time for the digestive tract to process red meat.

Tip 10:	**Eating Fruit with Meals**

Always eat your fruit first and then a full glass of water. Then eat your meal.

Tip 11:	**Alkaline pH**

Increase the alkaline content in your diet. To maintain optimal health the body fluids needs to be slightly alkaline.

Tip 12:	**Use Himalayan Salt**

The Himalayan Cooking Salt is the purest salt and contains the trace elements in their natural mineral form for the physical body needs.

Some of the benefits of Himalayan Salt:

- Helps with detoxification, which helps to regulate water content in the body.

- Supports the respiratory health.

- Helps to promote healthy blood sugar health.

- Healthy pH balance in your cells.

- Helps with the proper absorption of food particles in the digestive tract.

- Helps to promote healthy regulation of blood pressure.

Tip 13:	**Exercise**

Before each exercise use the activation and even during the exercise do the daily declarations. Get rid of the "sitting disease," being sedentary for more than 3 hours a day.

You need movement for at least 15 to 30 minutes.

- Walking for 15 - 30 minutes, ideally 7,000 to 10,000 steps daily. Go for a walk during your lunch break.
- Dancing around in your living space (find a fun line dance for 15 - 30 minutes)
- Jump roping at your own pace
- Bicycling is also good
- Swimming is a great exercise.
- Take a stretch break for at least 5 to 6 times a day.
- Take the stairs instead of the elevator.
- March in place or jog in place.

Try to be active most of the day; don't remain sedentary for more than 3 hours a day.

Tip 14:	**Fast**

To jumpstart your weight loss program and eating your way to a healthy lifestyle is to incorporate a "fast" to start the detoxification of your body. You can start by skipping breakfast, and eat your first meal at lunch. Do this to get rid of the sugar cravings and to boost your fat burning process. This will help your body burn fat instead of sugar.

Tip 15:	**Apps**

Use a pedometer app on your phone to count your steps/miles and duration when exercising. There are numerous tools to use: Fitbit and other fitness trackers to help monitor your activity.

Tip 16:	Eat organic, whole foods or locally grown.
Tip 17:	Eat smaller portions and to avoid overeating. Eat on "blue" plates. The color blue acts as an appetite suppressant
Tip 18:	Keep your digestive tract regular with regular bowel movements. Add a probiotic to your daily diet.

Tip 19:	**Liver Cleanse**

To cleanse your liver and to boost your metabolism, to fat
burn.

1 cup of hot water
½ lemon/lime
¼ turmeric
pinch of cayenne pepper
maple syrup, raw honey or stevia

Tip 20:	**Increase your Frequency** **Cut out the Coffee** **Cut out the** **processed/canned food** **[a]**

It has been discovered that everything has frequency. Our
body has a healthy daytime frequency of 62 to 68 Hz. It is
stated when the frequency drops our immune system is
compromised.

Coffee has been shown to drop the frequencies 8-12 hertz in a
matter of 3 seconds

Processed/canned food has zero frequency and may lower
healthy frequencies in the body.

So, how do you increase the frequency by eating healthy foods,
using the declarations, use of essential oils and music.
[b][c]

Tip 21:	**Essential Oils [d][e]**

The use of essential oils may be used to increase the
vibrational frequency levels in your body. The low
frequency oils helps support physical ailments, mid
frequency oils promote emotional change, and high
frequency oils encourage spiritual growth and relaxation.

Rose	320 MHz
Joy	189 MHz

Helichrysum	181 MHz
Thieves	150 MHz
Frankincense	147 MHz
Ravensara	134 MHz
Lavender	118 MHz
Myrrh	105 MHz
Blue Tansy	105 MHz
German Chamomile	105 MHz
Melissa	102 MHz
Juniper	98 MHz
Sandalwood	96 MHz
Citrus Fresh	91 MHz
Angelica	85 MHz
Peppermint	78 MHz
Galbanum	56 MHz
Basil	52 MHz
Purification	45 MHz

Tip 22:	**Beverages**

It is best for your digestive tract to drink your beverages room temperature. Drinking cold beverages shock and decrease the circulation in the stomach, intestinal tracts.

Tip 23:	**Test your Tap Water**

Another tool to use is a pH test strip to test your tap water before consumption. Also use to test your body's pH balance. May use water enhancers, pH drops and green drinks.

Tip 24:	**Green Tea or Herbal Tea**

Drink Green tea or herbal tea to help in the detox process.

4
FOODS TO EAT

Here's a collection of foods and food tips to help you eat your way to a healthy lifestyle. Enjoy!

Water: Drink mountain spring water and fresh spring water.

Juices: Drink juices from organic fruits

Sweeteners: Stevia, Ki Sweet

Spices: Use turmeric, cinnamon, ginger, cloves, cardamom, cayenne, garlic, black pepper, himalayan salt and dandelion.

Milk: Milks that are good for you are coconut milk, almond milk and coconut kefir.

Smoothies: Green Smoothies are highly recommended.

Proteins: Chicken Breast, Yogurt, Whey Protein,Whey Powder, Eggs poached, Eggs boiled

Vegetables: Eat organic, fresh or frozen. Use lots of green leafy vegetables, plus artichokes, asparagus, beets, broccoli, brussels sprouts, cabbage, carrots, cauliflower, celery, collard greens, corn, cucumbers, dandelions, eggplant, green beans, kale, leeks, lettuce, mushrooms, mustard greens, okra, onions, parsley, parsnips, peppers, potatoes, radishes, rutabagas, scallions, spinach, sprouts, squash, sweet potatoes, tomatoes, turnips, yams and zucchini.

Herbs: Use basil, bay leaves, cardamom, cayenne, chili powder, chives, cilantro (fresh coriander plant leaves), cinnamon, cloves, cumin, dill, garam masala, garlic, ginger, lemongrass, mint, mustard, nutmeg, oregano, paprika, parsley, black pepper, rosemary, sage, himalayan salt, sea salt, tarragon, thyme and turmeric.

Fruits: Use organic, fresh or frozen. Use apples, grapes, avocados, apricots, bananas, blackberries, blueberries, cantaloupe, cherries, coconuts, cranberries, dates, figs, grapefruit, guava, honeydew melons, kiwi, lemons, limes, mangoes, melons, nectarines, oranges, papayas, peaches, pineapples, plums, prunes, raisins, raspberries, strawberries, tangerines and watermelon.

A note here is to stay away from the sugary fruits or at least, use modest amounts.

Legumes: Eat pinto beans, lentils, black beans, black-eyed peas, kidney beans, mung beans and split peas.

Nuts: Eat shelled sunflower seeds, almonds, all nuts (raw, unsalted), including almonds, cashews, chia seeds, flaxseed, pumpkin seeds, sesame seeds, squash seeds, sunflower seeds and walnuts.

Grains: Use brown rice, quinoa, amaranth, barley, millet, oats (groats soaked - hulled or crushed grain).

Meats: Use ham hock as seasoning. Eat chicken and fish (baked or grilled). Eat red meat in moderation.

Snacks: Eat dried cranberries, almonds, apples, fresh coconut, raisins and dried dates.

Oils: Use avocado, canola, coconut, flaxseed, grape seed, peanut, olive oil, safflower oil, sesame oils and tahini.

ALKALINE versus ACIDIC FOODS

EAT MORE OF THESE		
Highly Alkaline Foods/Beverages	**Moderately Alkaline Foods/Beverages**	**Mildly Alkaline Foods/Beverages**
• Alfalfa Sprouts	• Arugula	• Almond Milk
• Broccoli	• Avocado	• Artichokes
• Cucumber	• Beetroot	• Asparagus
• Greens	• Butter Bean	• Avocado Oil
• Green drinks	• Capsicum/Pepper	• Beans & Legumes
• Kale	• Cabbage	• Brussels Sprouts
• Kelp	• Celery	• Buckwheat
• Parsley	• Chia Seeds	• Cauliflower

• Ph balanced 9.5 alkaline water	• Collard Greens	• Carrot
• Spinach	• Endive	• Chives
• Sprouts/Beans	• Garlic	• Coconut
	• Ginger	• Coconut Oil
	• Green Beans	• Flax Oil
	• Lemon	• Goat Milk
	• Lettuce	• Grapefruit
	• Lime	• Herbs & Spices
	• Mustard Greens	• Leeks
	• Okra	• Lentils
	• Quinoa	• New Baby Potatoes
	• Onion	• Peas
	• Radish	• Rhubarb
	• Red Onion	• Spelt
	• Soy Beans	• Swede
	• Tomato	• Tofu
	• White Haricot Beans	• Watercress

EAT LESS OF THESE – WATCH LIST

Mildly Acidic	Moderately Acidic	Highly Acidic
• Amaranth	• Apple	• Alcohol
• Black Beans	• Apricot	• Artificial Sweeteners
• Brazil Beans	• Banana	• Beef
• Chickpeas	• Blackberry	• Black Tea
• Cantaloupe	• Blueberry	• Cheese
• Currants	• Brown Rice	• Chicken
• Fresh Dates	• Butter	• Cocoa
• Fresh Water Wild Fish	• Cranberry	• Coffee
• Grape seed Oil	• Fresh, Natural Juice	• Dairy
• Hazel Nuts	• Grapes	• Dried Fruit
• Hemp Protein	• Ketchup	• Eggs
• Millet	• Mango	• Farmed Fish
• Nectarine	• Mangosteen	• Honey
• Oats/Oatmeal	• Mayonnaise	• Jam

• Pecan Nuts	• Oats	• Jelly
• Rice Milk	• Ocean Fish	• Miso
• Plum	• Orange	• Mushroom
• Rice Protein	• Peach	• Mustard
• Soy Milk	• Papaya	• Pork
• Soy Protein	• Pineapple	• Rice Syrup
• Soybeans	• Rye Bread	• Shellfish
• Spelt	• Strawberry	• Soy Sauce
• Sunflower Oil	• Wheat	• Syrup
• Sweet Cherry	• Wholemeal Bread	• Vinegar
• Watermelon	• Wild Rice	• Yeast
	• Wholemeal Pasta	

5
SAMPLE MEAL PLANS

Before starting the sample meal plans, I recommend a 3 day liver detox, to cleanse and strengthen the liver and gallbladder function. Use the liver detox recipe in the Tips Section. In some cases, it takes longer for the liver to be cleansed if need be, do a cleanse for 21 days. You want that your liver is not being overworked.

I also recommend a colon cleanse as well to cleanse the gastrointestinal system. Another recommendation is to do this for 21 days consistently so you can receive the results and change your mindset about eating. This is a process of changing your old way into a healthy lifestyle of eating. Make sure always to consult your physician before starting any plan.

This is not a quick fix or a bandage; this is a transformation from the inside out. I encourage you to continue and push through when you want to go back to what is convenient or just say to yourself "this is too hard". I say to you, right now "LIVE". I need you to live. Your family needs you to live. You must live to fulfill your "DESTINY". What you was created to be, do and fulfill. Therefore, everyday ask, "Have I completed my destiny", "What I am called to do", and then I must continue through the pain and the flesh wanting its desires.

It is recommended that you eat 6 meals a day. Be mindful of the portions. These are light portions. The below sample meal plan is what I setup for myself. However, I recommend that you may use it as a guide really to keep of time management to eat for fuel for the body to function properly throughout the day. There is a Daily Journal in the next section for you to track your day. Following that section are simple recipes to kick start your process. Just be patient and be encouraged as you start this. Remember, what I stated earlier about the foods that I wasn't accustomed to eating, the Lord said I would begin to enjoy as my body detoxify from the old way. This is new day, new life's journey as you continue to launch forward.

Sample Meal Plans

1st Day	
Upon arising, drink full glass of warm water to flush system.	
6:00 AM – Breakfast	Oatmeal Nuts & Fruit Cup, 1 serving Greens Smoothie, 8 oz.
7:00 AM - 8:00 AM	Drink Apple Cider Vinegar, 8 oz. glass
9:00 AM - Snack	Almonds, 1 1/2 teaspoons
10:00 AM – 11:00 AM	Drink Apple Cider Vinegar, 8 oz. glass
12:00 PM - Lunch	Grilled Chicken Breast, 2oz Asparagus, 4 spears Roasted Vegetables, 1/2 cup
1:00 PM – 2:00 PM	Drink Apple Cider Vinegar, 8 oz glass

3:00 PM - Snack	Apple slices with peanut butter
4:00 PM – 5:00 PM	Drink Lemon/Lime Water , 8 oz glass
6:00 PM - Dinner	Grilled Salmon, 1 serving Spinach Salad, 1 cup Stir Fry String Beans, 1/2 cup
7:00 PM – 8:00 PM	Drink Lemon/Lime Water, 8 oz glass
9:00 PM - Snack	1 cup of red grapes, 1 cup
Make sure you try to drink 8 glasses of water daily	
2nd Day	
Upon arising, drink full glass of warm water to flush system.	
6:00 AM – Breakfast	Juicy Juice Smoothie, 8 oz Herbal Tea or Green Tea, 1 cup
7:00 AM - 8:00 AM	Drink Apple Cider Vinegar, 8 oz glass
9:00 AM - Snack	Tuna Salad on Apples, 4-6 slices
10:00 AM – 11:00 AM	Drink Apple Cider Vinegar, 8 oz glass
12:00 PM - Lunch	Garden Turkey Burger, 2 oz Lentil Soup, 1/2 cup
1:00 PM – 2:00 PM	Drink Apple Cider Vinegar, 8 oz glass
3:00 PM - Snack	Orange, 1 cup sections
4:00 PM – 5:00 PM	Drink Lemon/Lime Water, 8 oz glass
6:00 PM - Dinner	Cool Cucumber Spinach Herb Wrap, 3 oz Strawberry Salad, 1 cup
7:00 PM – 8:00 PM	Drink Lemon/Lime Water, 8 oz glass
9:00 PM - Snack	Hummus with carrot sticks, 3 oz
Make sure you try to drink 8 glasses of water daily	
3rd Day	
Upon arising, drink full glass of warm water to flush system.	
6:00 AM – Breakfast	Carrot Juice, 8 oz glass Breakfast Omelet, 1 serving Herbal Tea or Green Tea, 1 cup
7:00 AM - 8:00 AM	Drink Apple Cider Vinegar, 8 oz glass
9:00 AM - Snack	Hard boiled Eggs, 1 or 2
10:00 AM – 11:00 AM	Drink Apple Cider Vinegar, 8 oz glass
12:00 PM - Lunch	Grilled Chicken Salad, 1 serving Carrot Soup, 1 cup

1:00 PM – 2:00 PM	Drink Apple Cider Vinegar, 8 oz glass
3:00 PM - Snack	Cup of Blueberries, 1 serving
4:00 PM – 5:00 PM	Drink Lemon/Lime Water, 8 oz glass
6:00 PM - Dinner	Carrots & Broccoli, 1/2 cup Roasted Vegetables, 1/2 cup Grilled Salmon, 1 serving
7:00 PM – 8:00 PM	Drink Lemon/Lime Water , 8 oz glass
9:00 PM - Snack	Broccoli with Hummus, 2 oz
Make sure you try to drink 8 glasses of water daily	
4th Day	
Upon arising, drink full glass of warm water to flush system.	
6:00 AM – Breakfast	2 scrambled eggs, 1 serving turkey bacon, 2 strips Green tea, 1 cup Kale, Banana & Strawberry Smoothie, 8 oz glass
7:00 AM - 8:00 AM	Drink Apple Cider Vinegar, 8 oz glass
9:00 AM - Snack	Baked Sweet Potato, 1 serving
10:00 AM – 11:00 AM	Drink Apple Cider Vinegar, 8 oz glass
12:00 PM - Lunch	Jerk Chicken Nachos, 1 serving
1:00 PM – 2:00 PM	Drink Apple Cider Vinegar, 8 oz glass
3:00 PM - Snack	Banana, 1 whole
4:00 PM – 5:00 PM	Drink Lemon/Lime Water, 8 oz glass
6:00 PM - Dinner	Fruit Cup (Eat fruit first), 1 cup Chicken Lettuce Wraps, 1 serving
7:00 PM – 8:00 PM	Drink Lemon/Lime Water, 8 oz glass
9:00 PM - Snack	Carrots & cucumber sticks, 16 sticks
Make sure you try to drink 8 glasses of water daily	
5th Day	
Upon arising, drink full glass of warm water to flush system.	
6:00 AM – Breakfast	Breakfast Egg Muffin, 1 serving Herbal Tea or Green Tea, 1 cup Green Apple Smoothie, 8 oz glass
7:00 AM - 8:00 AM	Drink Apple Cider Vinegar, 8 oz glass
9:00 AM - Snack	Tuna Stuffed Cucumbers, 2 servings
10:00 AM – 11:00 AM	Drink Apple Cider Vinegar, 8 oz glass

12:00 PM - Lunch	Grilled Chicken Breast, 1 serving Asparagus, 5 spears	
1:00 PM – 2:00 PM	Drink Apple Cider Vinegar, 8 oz glass	
3:00 PM - Snack	Baked Potato, 1 whole	
4:00 PM – 5:00 PM	Drink Lemon/Lime Water , 8 oz glass	
6:00 PM - Dinner	Carrot Soup, 1/2 cup Roasted Vegetables, 1/2 cup Grilled Salmon, 1 serving	
7:00 PM – 8:00 PM	Drink Lemon/Lime Water	8 oz. glass
9:00 PM - Snack	Apple slices with peanut butter	
Make sure you try to drink 8 glasses of water daily		
6th Day		
Upon arising, drink full glass of warm water to flush system.		
6:00 AM – Breakfast	Grapefruit w/yogurt, 1 serving Hard Boiled Egg, 1 egg Green Tea, 1 cup	
7:00 AM - 8:00 AM	Drink Apple Cider Vinegar, 8 oz glass	
9:00 AM - Snack	Broccoli with Hummus, 2 oz	
10:00 AM – 11:00 AM	Drink Apple Cider Vinegar, 8 oz glass	
12:00 PM - Lunch	Garden Turkey Burger, 2 oz Lentil Soup, 1/2 cup	
1:00 PM – 2:00 PM	Drink Apple Cider Vinegar, 8 oz glass	
3:00 PM - Snack	Orange, 1 whole	
4:00 PM – 5:00 PM	Drink Lemon/Lime Water, 8 oz glass	
6:00 PM - Dinner	Cool Cucumber Spinach Herb Wrap, 1 serving Strawberry Salad, 1 cup	
7:00 PM – 8:00 PM	Drink Lemon/Lime Water, 8 oz glass	
9:00 PM - Snack	1 cup of red grapes, 1 cup	
Make sure you try to drink 8 glasses of water daily		
7th Day		
Upon arising, drink full glass of warm water to flush system.		
6:00 AM – Breakfast	Breakfast Omelet, 1 omelet Strawberry, Peach, Banana Split Smoothie, 8 oz glass	

7:00 AM - 8:00 AM	Drink Apple Cider Vinegar, 8 oz glass
9:00 AM - Snack	Skinny Popcorn with Chia Seeds, Granola, Coconut & Almonds, 1 cup
10:00 AM – 11:00 AM	Drink Apple Cider Vinegar, 8 oz glass
12:00 PM - Lunch	Chicken Lettuce Wraps, 1 serving
1:00 PM – 2:00 PM	Drink Apple Cider Vinegar, 8 oz glass
3:00 PM - Snack	Fruit Cup, 1 cup
4:00 PM – 5:00 PM	Drink Lemon/Lime Water, 8 oz glass
6:00 PM - Dinner	Jerk Chicken Nachos, 1 serving
7:00 PM – 8:00 PM	Drink Lemon/Lime Water, 8 oz glass
9:00 PM - Snack	Tuna Stuffed Cucumbers, 2 servings
Make sure you try to drink 8 glasses of water daily	

6
DAILY MEAL PLAN JOURNAL

Day 1- *My soul shall be satisfied as with marrow and fatness; and my mouth shall praise thee with joyful lips:* **Psalm 63:5**

Breakfast____

Snack____

Lunch____

Snack____

Dinner____

Snack____

Water Consumption: _____________________________________

Write how you felt during the

day.____

____

____

Any physical effects (like headaches, dizziness,

etc)____

Daily Exercise:____

Notes for today:

____

____

____

____

____

Day 2 - *A sound heart is the life of the flesh: but envy the rottenness of the bones.* Proverbs 14:30

Breakfast____

Snack____

Lunch____

Snack____

Dinner____

Snack____

Water Consumption: ___________________________________

Write how you felt during the

day.___________________________________

____

____

Any physical effects (like headaches, dizziness,

etc)___________________________________

Daily Exercise:___________________________________

Notes for today:

____

____

____

____

____

***Day 3**- But refuse profane and old wives' fables, and exercise thyself rather unto godliness. 8 For bodily exercise profiteth little: but godliness is profitable unto all things, having promise of the life that now is, and of that which is to come. 9 This is a faithful saying and worthy of all acceptation. 1 Timothy 4:7-9*

Breakfast___________________________________

Snack___________________________________

Lunch___________________________________

Snack___________________________________

Dinner___________________________________

Snack___________________________________

Water Consumption: ___________________________________

Write how you felt during the

day.___________________________________

____

____

Any physical effects (like headaches, dizziness,

etc)___________________________________

Daily Exercise:___________________________________

Notes for today:

____

____

____
____
____
____

Day 4- *[16] Know ye not that ye are the temple of God, and that the Spirit of God dwelleth in you? [17] If any man defile the temple of God, him shall God destroy; for the temple of God is holy, which temple ye are.* *1 Corinthians 3:16-17*

Breakfast____
Snack____
Lunch____
Snack____
Dinner____
Snack____
Water Consumption: _____________________________________
Write how you felt during the
day.____
____
____

Any physical effects (like headaches, dizziness,
etc)____
Daily Exercise: ____
Notes for today:

____
____
____
____
____

Day 5- *[19] What? know ye not that your body is the temple of the Holy Ghost which is in you, which ye have of God, and ye are not your own? [20] For ye are bought with a price: therefore glorify God in your body, and in your spirit, which are God's.* *1 Corinthians 6:19-20*

Breakfast____
Snack____
Lunch____
Snack____

Dinner____

Snack____

Water Consumption: _________________________________

Write how you felt during the

day.____

____

____

Any physical effects (like headaches, dizziness,

etc)____

Daily Exercise:______________________________________

Notes for today:

____

____

____

____

____

Day 6 - 12 *I beseech you therefore, brethren, by the mercies of God, that ye present your bodies a living sacrifice, holy, acceptable unto God, which is your reasonable service. 2 And be not conformed to this world: but be ye transformed by the renewing of your mind, that ye may prove what is that good, and acceptable, and perfect, will of God.* ***Romans 12:1-2***

Breakfast____

Snack____

Lunch____

Snack____

Dinner____

Snack____

Water Consumption: _________________________________

Write how you felt during the

day.____

____

____

Any physical effects (like headaches, dizziness,

etc)____

Daily Exercise: _____________________________________

Notes for today:

____
____
____
____
____
____

Day 7- *7 Be not wise in thine own eyes: fear the LORD, and depart from evil. 8 It shall be health to thy navel, and marrow to thy bones.* Proverbs 3:7-8

Breakfast_______________________________________

Snack_______________________________________

Lunch_______________________________________

Snack_______________________________________

Dinner_______________________________________

Snack_______________________________________

Water Consumption: _______________________________

Write how you felt during the

day._______________________________________
____
____

Any physical effects (like headaches, dizziness,

etc)_______________________________________

Daily Exercise: _______________________________

Notes for today:

____
____
____
____
____

Day 8- *28 Come unto me, all ye that labour and are heavy laden, and I will give you rest. 29 Take my yoke upon you, and learn of me; for I am meek and lowly in heart: and ye shall find rest unto your souls.* Matthew 11:28-29

Breakfast_______________________________________

Snack_______________________________________

Lunch_______________________________________

Snack_______________________________________

Dinner_______________________________________

Snack____
Water Consumption: _________________________________
Write how you felt during the
day.____

____

Any physical effects (like headaches, dizziness,
etc)____
Daily Exercise: _____________________________________
Notes for today:

____

____

____

____

____

Day 9- *29 He giveth power to the faint; and to them that have no might he increaseth strength. 30 Even the youths shall faint and be weary, and the young men shall utterly fall: 31 But they that wait upon the LORD shall renew their strength; they shall mount up with wings as eagles; they shall run, and not be weary; and they shall walk, and not faint. Isaiah 40:29-31*
Breakfast____
Snack____
Lunch____
Snack____
Dinner____
Snack____
Water Consumption: _________________________________
Write how you felt during the
day.____

____

Any physical effects (like headaches, dizziness,
etc)____
Daily Exercise: _____________________________________
Notes for today:

____

____
____
____
____
____
____

Day 10 - *8 But meat commendeth us not to God: for neither, if we eat, are we the better; neither, if we eat not, are we the worse. 1 Corinthians 8:8*

Breakfast_________________________________
Snack____________________________________
Lunch____________________________________
Snack____________________________________
Dinner___________________________________
Snack____________________________________
Water Consumption: _______________________
Write how you felt during the
day.______________________________________

____

Any physical effects (like headaches, dizziness,
etc)______________________________________
Daily Exercise: ___________________________
Notes for today:

____
____
____
____
____

Day 11- *15 The eyes of all wait upon thee; and thou givest them their meat in due season. 16 Thou openest thine hand, and satisfiest the desire of every living thing. Psalm 145:15-16*

Breakfast_________________________________
Snack____________________________________
Lunch____________________________________
Snack____________________________________
Dinner___________________________________
Snack____________________________________

Water Consumption: _______________________________________
Write how you felt during the
day.____

____

Any physical effects (like headaches, dizziness,
etc)____
Daily Exercise: ____
Notes for today:

____

____

____

____

____

Day 12 *- Ho, every one that thirsteth, come ye to the waters, and he that hath no money; come ye, buy, and eat; yea, come, buy wine and milk without money and without price. ²Wherefore do ye spend money for that which is not bread? and your labour for that which satisfieth not? hearken diligently unto me, and eat ye that which is good, and let your soul delight itself in fatness.* *Isaiah 55: 1-2*

Breakfast____
Snack____
Lunch____
Snack____
Dinner____
Snack____
Water Consumption: _______________________________________
Write how you felt during the
day.____

____

Any physical effects (like headaches, dizziness,
etc)____
Daily Exercise: ____
Notes for today:

____

____
____
____
____
____

Day 13- [11] *And the LORD shall guide thee continually, and satisfy thy soul in drought, and make fat thy bones: and thou shalt be like a watered garden, and like a spring of water, whose waters fail not. Isaiah 58:11*

Breakfast_______________________________________

Snack_______________________________________

Lunch_______________________________________

Snack_______________________________________

Dinner_______________________________________

Snack_______________________________________

Water Consumption: _______________________________

Write how you felt during the

day._______________________________________

____

Any physical effects (like headaches, dizziness,

etc)_______________________________________

Daily Exercise: _______________________________

Notes for today:

____
____
____
____
____

Day 14- [93] *I will never forget thy precepts: for with them thou hast quickened me. Psalm 119: 93*

Breakfast_______________________________________

Snack_______________________________________

Lunch_______________________________________

Snack_______________________________________

Dinner_______________________________________

Snack_______________________________________

Water Consumption: _______________________________________
Write how you felt during the
day.____

____

Any physical effects (like headaches, dizziness,
etc)____
Daily Exercise: ____
Notes for today:

____
____
____
____
____

Day 15- [22] *A merry heart doeth good like a medicine: but a broken spirit drieth the bones.* Proverbs 17:22
Breakfast____
Snack____
Lunch____
Snack____
Dinner____
Snack____
Water Consumption: _______________________________________
Write how you felt during the
day.____

____

Any physical effects (like headaches, dizziness,
etc)____
Daily Exercise: ____
Notes for today:

____
____
____
____
____

Day 16- *²⁵ And ye shall serve the LORD your God, and he shall bless thy bread, and thy water; and I will take sickness away from the midst of thee.* Exodus 23:25

Breakfast____

Snack____

Lunch____

Snack____

Dinner____

Snack____

Water Consumption: ______________________________________

Write how you felt during the

day.____

____

Any physical effects (like headaches, dizziness,

etc)____

Daily Exercise: ____

Notes for today:

____

____

____

____

____

Day 17- *²⁵ And ye shall serve the LORD your God, and he shall bless thy bread, and thy water; and I will take sickness away from the midst of thee.* Psalm 28:7

Breakfast____

Snack____

Lunch____

Snack____

Dinner____

Snack____

Water Consumption: ______________________________________

Write how you felt during the

day.____

Any physical effects (like headaches, dizziness, etc)____
Daily Exercise: _______________________________________
Notes for today:

____
____
____
____
____

Day 18- [143] *Trouble and anguish have taken hold on me: yet thy commandments are my delights.* Psalm 119:143
Breakfast____
Snack____
Lunch____
Snack____
Dinner____
Snack____
Water Consumption: ________________________________
Write how you felt during the day.____

____
____

Any physical effects (like headaches, dizziness, etc)____
Daily Exercise: _______________________________________
Notes for today:

____
____
____
____
____

Day 19- [6] *Be careful for nothing; but in every thing by prayer and supplication with thanksgiving let your requests be made known unto God.* [7] *And the peace* *of God, which passeth all understanding, shall keep your hearts and minds through Christ Jesus.* Philippians 4:6-7

Breakfast____

Snack____

Lunch____

Snack____

Dinner____

Snack____

Water Consumption: ______________________________________

Write how you felt during the

day.____

____

____

Any physical effects (like headaches, dizziness,

etc)____

Daily Exercise: ____

Notes for today:

____

____

____

____

____

Day 20- [31] *Whether therefore ye eat, or drink, or whatsoever ye do, do all to the glory of God.* 1 Corinthians 10:31

Breakfast____

Snack____

Lunch____

Snack____

Dinner____

Snack____

Water Consumption: ______________________________________

Write how you felt during the

day.____

____

____

Any physical effects (like headaches, dizziness,

etc)____

Daily Exercise: _______________________________________

Notes for today:

____

____

____

____

____

Day 21 - [2] *Beloved, I wish above all things that thou mayest prosper and be in health, even as thy soul prospereth.* 3 John 2

Breakfast____

Snack____

Lunch____

Snack____

Dinner____

Snack____

Water Consumption: ______________________________

Write how you felt during the

day.____

____

Any physical effects (like headaches, dizziness,

etc)____

Daily Exercise: _______________________________________

Notes for today:

____

____

____

____

____

7
RECIPES

These recipes are light fare that can be made very quickly and are very healthy. Substitutions can be made as well.

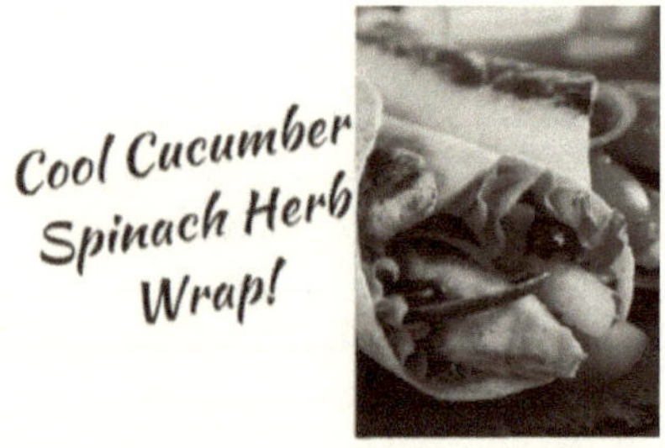

Ingredients

Makes 1-2 Servings
2 Spinach Herb Wrap already made
½ cup chopped tomatoes
¼ cup chopped sweet Vidalia onions
½ cup chopped cucumbers without seeds
1 sprig of fresh cilantro chopped
½ cup of black beans
1 cup of fresh spring mix salad or fresh spinach
1-cup sautéed chicken breast strips
Ranch Dressing or Cool Cucumber Dressing

Preparation

Layer all the ingredients on the spinach herb wrap. Then add the cilantro and dressing. Then roll up the wrap.

Cool Cucumber Dressing
1 packet of ranch dressing
1 large cucumber, peeled, seeded and chopped
pinch of salt
pinch of ground peppercorn
½ cup of sour cream
Add 1 Tablespoon of Extra Virgin Olive Oil

Preparation
Combine the ingredients in a blender or food processor. Cover and blend until creamy and smooth. Put in container covered and chill. Serve over your wrap, salad or use as a dip.

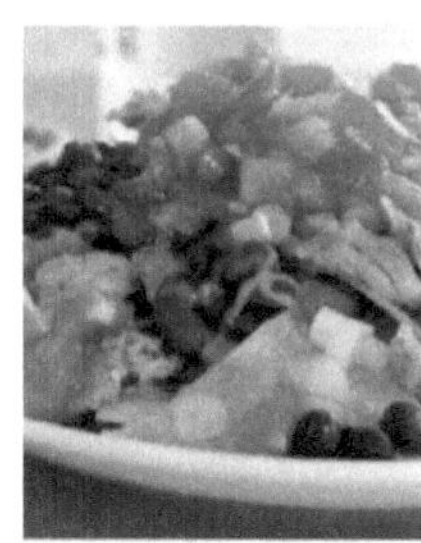

Jerk Chicken Nachos!

Ingredients

Makes 1-2 Servings
2 multi-grain nacho chips
1 cup chopped tomatoes

2 tablespoons fresh cilantro chopped
1 cup black beans, cooked and drained
1 large peeled, seeded, chopped cucumber
1/2 cup whole sweet kernel corn, drained
2 cups fresh spring mix salad
jalapeño peppers
Jerk Chicken (see recipe below)

Preparation

In a large plate or platter, pour and spread out the multi-grain nachos. Layer over the nachos, the fresh spring mix salad, jerk chicken mixture, black beans, sweet kernel corn, chopped tomatoes, cucumbers, fresh cilantro, jalapeno peppers. May add sour cream or salsa to this dish if you desire.

Jerk Chicken

2 chicken breast cut into small pieces
McCormick Jerk Seasoning
1 cup chopped sweet vidalia onions
1 cup of red, yellow and green bell peppers (optional)
Jerk sauce and marinade
red pepper flakes (optional)
1 Tablespoon stir-fry oil

Preparation

Marinate the chicken breast in the jerk sauce and marinate overnight.

In a large frying pan or wok add stir-fry oil. Add the chicken and cook until done. Add the onions, red, yellow and green peppers until vegetables are cooked. Add the McCormick Jerk Seasoning to taste. Set aside.

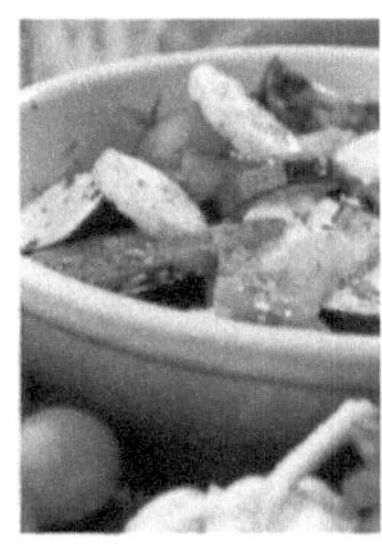

Submitted by: Fatima Lansana
Ingredients

1 Zucchini, sliced and quartered
1 Yellow squash, sliced and quartered
2 cups mushrooms
2 cups broccoli florets
3 Bell Peppers, seeded and diced (red, yellow, orange)
2 Tomatoes, sliced and quartered

2 Red onions, quartered
2 cups cauliflower
2 tablespoons Olive oil
4 cloves garlic, minced
1 1/2 teaspoons Dried thyme
Black pepper to taste

Himalayan Salt to taste
Balsamic vinegar

Other vegetables you can add or substitute: fresh string beans, asparagus, sweet potatoes, yams, and Brussels sprouts.

Preparation

Preheat oven to 400 degrees F. (Temperature may vary depending on your stove)
Spray pan with non-stick spray or coat lightly with oil.

Slice up vegetables and place them in a large bowl or container. You may also place them in a large zip lock bag to toss them with the rest of the ingredients.

Add minced garlic, thyme, salt, black pepper, olive oil and balsamic vinegar to vegetables and mix until they are all coated. Let this mixture marinate for at least 15-20 minutes to allow flavors to soak in to vegetables.

Lay veggies out on a tray and roast in oven for about 20-25 minutes. You can do less if you prefer crunchy veggies or a little more if you prefer softer veggies.

Adjust the seasoning to your taste. You can add more balsamic vinegar as well.

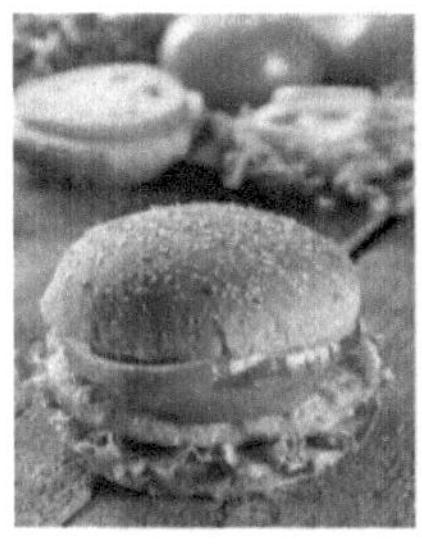

Garden Turkey Burger!

Ingredients

Makes 1-2 Servings

1-pound fresh ground turkey
1 small red onion, sliced into rings
½ pouch of ranch onion dip mix
1 small tomato, sliced
bunch of spinach leaves
Jalapeño Peppers
Condiments of choice
toasted slider buns

Preparation

Preheat grill to medium-high.

Combine the ground turkey and ranch onion dip mix thoroughly. Form 3-6 burgers.

Oil the grill rack and grill the burgers are cooked medium well, 2-3 minutes on each side.

Toast the buns and then assemble with condiments of your choice (mayonnaise, mustard), spinach leaves, onion, tomato, jalapeno peppers.

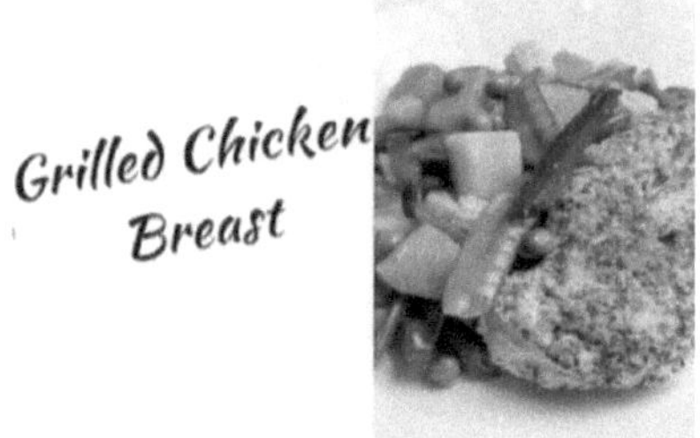

Ingredients
Makes 2 servings
2 boneless skinless chicken breasts (make sure skin is removed)
2 teaspoons of spicy seasoned salt
2 tablespoons extra virgin olive oil (EVOO)
lemon slices

Preparation

Preheat grill on high for about 5 minutes. Properly oil the grill to ensure cleanliness of the grill.

Drill the olive oil over the chicken breasts and seasoned with spicy seasoned salt. Place the chicken on the grill and cook covered for 4-5 minutes on both sides. Make sure chicken is thoroughly cooked with no pink color.

May serve on a bed of brown rice, and mixed fresh greens. Can plate with roasted vegetables, asparagus and chicken breast. Squeeze lemon on chicken and serve.

Spicy Seasoned Salt

2 tablespoons chili powder

3 tablespoons of paprika

1 tablespoon of ground red pepper flakes

3 tablespoons of ground black peppercorn

¼ cup garlic powder

¼ cup onion powder

3 tablespoons of dried parsley leaves

Mix all ingredients in a mason jar and shake. Maybe placed in a food processor to blend finely. Store in sealed, airtight mason jar.

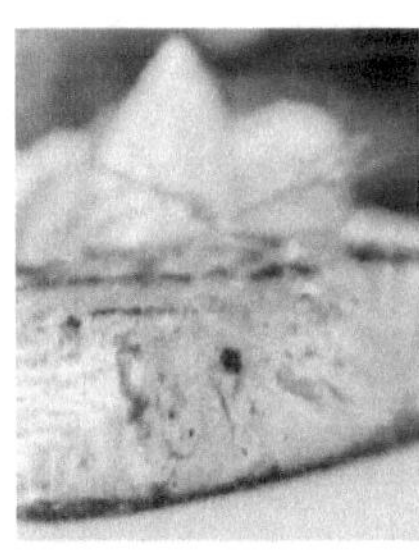

Grilled Salmon!

Ingredients

Makes 2 servings

2 salmon fillets

sea salt and ground pepper to taste

½ cup mayonnaise
1-tablespoon fresh squeezed lemon juice
2 tablespoons extra virgin olive oil
2 tablespoons Dijon mustard
4 garlic cloves, minced
¼ teaspoon ground black pepper
¼ teaspoon sea salt
2 tablespoons chopped fresh tarragon

Preparation

Preheat grill on high for about 5 minutes. Properly oil the grill to ensure cleanliness of the grill. Lightly oil the grill grate to make sure the salmon doesn't stick.

Season the salmon with salt and pepper on both sides. Drizzle with olive oil on both sides.

Now whisk the following: Dijon mustard, mayonnaise, olive oil, garlic, lemon juice, tarragon, salt and pepper. Set aside the sauce for serving over the salmon.

Place the salmon on the grill until the salmon flakes after 5-10 minutes. Plate the salmon and top with the sauce.

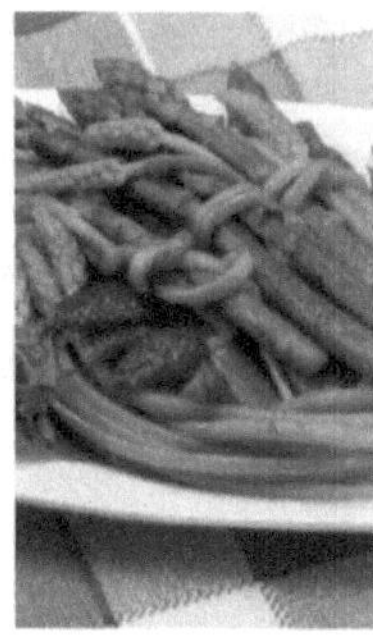

Ingredients

Makes 1-2 servings
Bunch of fresh asparagus spears
¼ teaspoon of sea salt
1 teaspoon of butter
1.5 cups of water
1.5 cups of chicken or vegetable stock
minced garlic (optional)
slices of lime

Preparation

Trim off the dry ends of the asparagus. Asparagus may need to be peeled according to the thickness. Use a vegetable peeler to peel them lightly. Set aside.

In a steamer pan set, add the water, garlic and broth and bring to a hard boil. Now place the asparagus on top of the steamer pan and let it steam for 5 to 10 minutes depending on the thickness of the asparagus or until tender. Just before serving, squeeze lime slice over the asparagus for more of a kick.

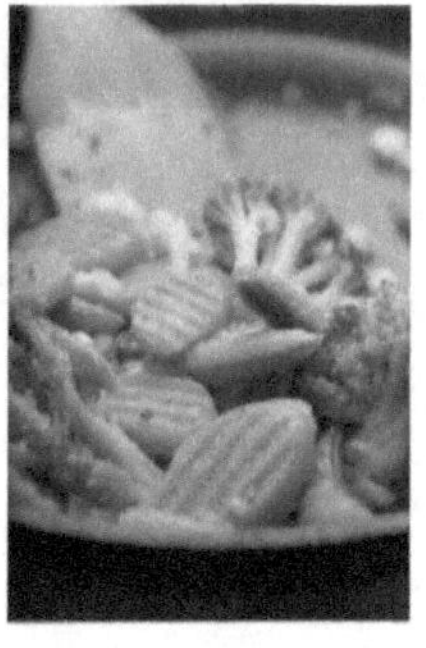

Carrot &
Broccoli
Stir Fry

Ingredients

Make 2 servings
1 teaspoon of vegetable broth
1 chicken bouillon cube, crushed or use granules.
6 cups of broccoli florets
1 carrot, sliced
1-teaspoon cornstarch
2 tablespoons stir fry oil
salt to taste

Preparation

In a large pot of salted water bring to a boil, add the broccoli and cook until green, about 1 minute now add the sliced carrots, cooked for 1 minute. Then drain. Blanche the broccoli and carrots in a bathe of ice water to stop the cooking process and drain.

Mix the cornstarch, vegetable broth until smooth. Now add the chicken bouillon and salt and mix well

In a heated wok add the stir-fry oil, add the vegetables and sauté for 2 minutes and the add the cornstarch mixture and cooked for 2 minutes. Make sure the vegetables are well coated evenly.

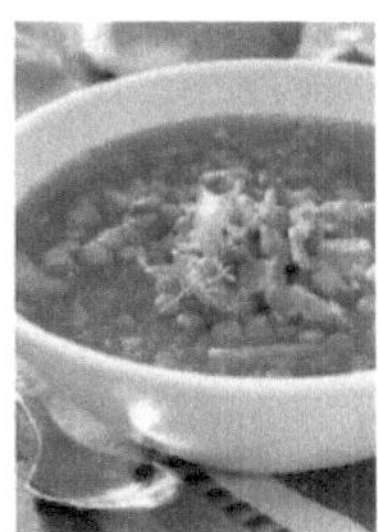

Ingredients

2 cups lentils
1-cup pinto beans
1 ham hock or ham bone
4 cups water
4 cups chicken or vegetable broth
or 8 cups chicken or vegetable broth
3 bouillon cubes (add additional for your taste)
½ onion chopped
whole bay leaf
1 cup chopped celery
1 cup green bell pepper
1 teaspoon dried marjoram

salt to taste
for added kick – red pepper flakes
black pepper to taste

Preparation

Before cooking the lentils rinse in cold water and remove any debris and drain. You can soak them as well to reduce cooking time.

Let the pinto beans soak overnight and make sure they are thoroughly cleansed.

Bring water, broth, and bouillon cubes to a boil in a stock pot and stirring to dissolve the bouillon cubes. Add the ham hock or ham bone to the pot and reduce the heat to medium. Add the pinto beans and let cook until beans are almost completely cooked. Then add the lentils and cook for about 10 minutes.

Add in the onions, celery, green bell pepper, bay leaf, marjoram, salt, red pepper flakes, and black pepper and bring to a simmer until beans, lentils and vegetables are tender, about 10 to 25 minutes.

Remove from heat and cut up the ham bone meat or ham hock and add to soup. Throw away the bone.

Before serving remove the bay leaf. Add a sprig of mint or parsley on top. May also added a little sour cream on top.

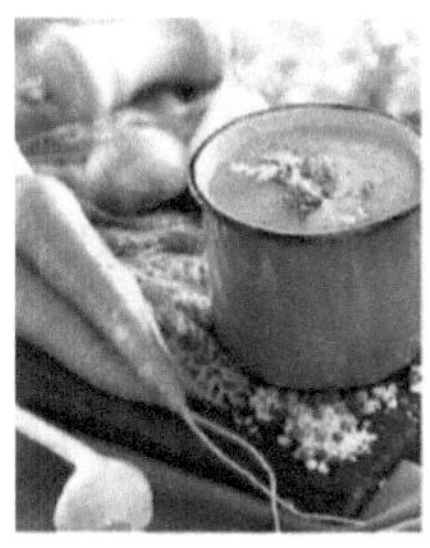

Carrot Soup

Ingredients

Makes 4-6 servings
3 pounds carrots, chopped
1 tablespoon extra virgin olive oil
3 cloves garlic, chopped
1 fresh red chile pepper, chopped
2 large onions, chopped
1 can roma tomatoes, with juice
2 cups vegetable stock or broth
1 bunch chopped fresh cilantro
1 ½ teaspoons sea salt
2 tablespoons balsamic vinegar
1 tablespoon sugar
ground black pepper to taste
1 cup whole milk

Preparation

Heat the olive oil in a large pot over medium heat and add the onions, carrots, chile pepper, garlic until tender.

Mix in the vegetable stock or broth, tomatoes, balsamic vinegar, sugar and ½ cilantro. Season this mixture with salt and pepper and bring to a boil. Reduce the heat to low and simmer for 30 minutes.

After the soup has cooked for the 30 minutes, add the soup to blender in separate batches and blend until smooth. Return soup into pot after blending and cook until heated thoroughly. Now remove from heat and add the milk slowly to the soup. Now add the remaining cilantro either to the soup or serve on top of each bowl of soup. Serve. May add some pita bread or flat bread.

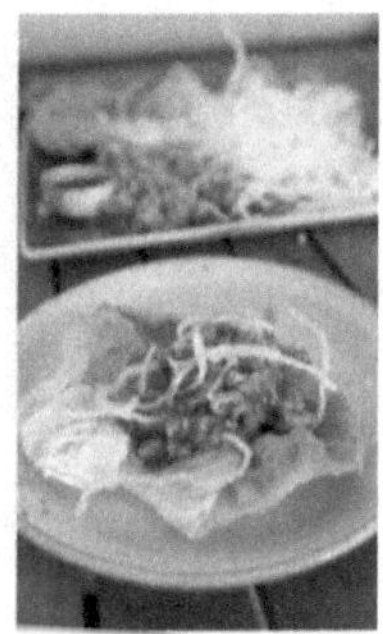

Chicken Lettuce Wraps

Ingredients

1 lb. ground chicken or 1 lb. ground turkey
½ cup fresh cilantro

2 cloves, garlic
2 green scallions, finely chopped
1 onion chopped
1 tablespoon freshly grated ginger
Large pieces of lettuce or butter lettuce
1 teaspoon sea salt
1 teaspoon ground black pepper
2 teaspoon sugar
¼ cup hoisin sauce
1 tablespoon olive oil
1 tablespoon rice wine vinegar
May use spinach wraps instead of lettuce

Preparation

Heat pan or wok with olive oil over medium high heat, then add 1 lb. ground chicken, let it brown and cook thoroughly. Drain the excess fat.

Add the following onions, rice wine vinegar, ginger, and hoisin sauce until onions become translucent for 2-3 minutes.

Stir in the scallions until tender and season with salt and pepper, to taste.

Serve with lettuce and your choice of condiments, but not necessary. Roll up in lettuce and enjoy.

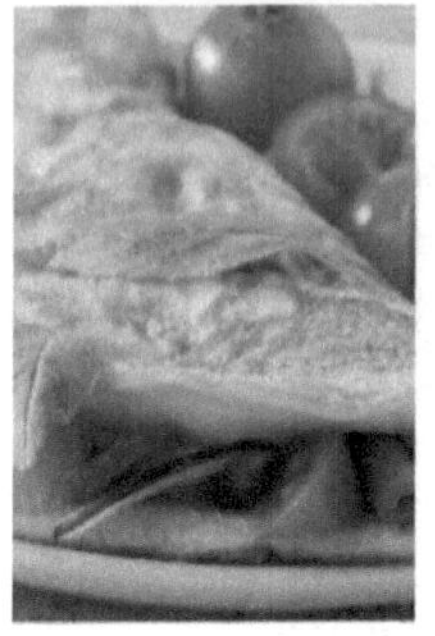

Breakfast Omelette!

Ingredients

2 large organic eggs
¼ cup red, yellow, green bell peppers, diced
¼ cup onions, diced
1 small tomato, diced
2 sprigs of fresh basil, chopped
sea salt
fresh ground black pepper
olive oil

Preparation

In a 8-inch nonstick skillet, heat oil over medium-high heat. Add the bell pepper and onions. Cook until onions are tender for about 2 minutes. Stir mixture. Remove the mixture from pan, set aside.

Now, pick the leaves off of the basil and tear them. You may chopped if you desire. Dice the tomato. Set this aside as well.

In a medium bowl, crack the eggs and add a dash of salt and pepper. Beat the eggs with fork until well mixed.

Now in the same skillet heat over medium heat with oil and quickly pour in the egg mixture into the pan. Tilt the pan to spread them out evenly.

Use a fork to swirl the eggs and let the eggs cook until they thicken. Let the omelette lightly brown. Do not overcook.

Slide the omelette onto plate and add the onion and bell peppers, basil on half of the omelette and fold. To taste add salt and black pepper. Serve immediately. Enjoy. Garnish basil leaves.

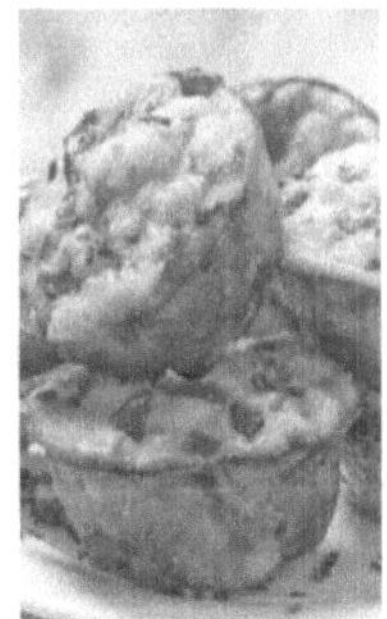

Ingredients

Ground turkey sausage cooked and crumbled
1 cup tomatoes, diced

1 cup sweet bell peppers
½ cup diced onions
1 cup fresh chopped spinach
1 dozen eggs
Salt and pepper to taste
1 tablespoon of olive oil
salsa (optional)

Preparation

Preheat oven to 350 degrees F. Spray non-stick muffin pan with nonstick spray. Sautee bell pepper and onions for 2-3 minutes. Stir in the spinach and sausage and let cook for 2 minutes.

Now add a tablespoon full into each muffin cup, and add the tomatoes.
Whisk the eggs in a medium bowl add salt and pepper to taste and pour the mixture over the sausage mixture in the muffin pan. Do not fill cup completely.

Place in oven and cook for about 25 minutes or until toothpick comes out clean.

May serve with a dollop of salsa and avocado.

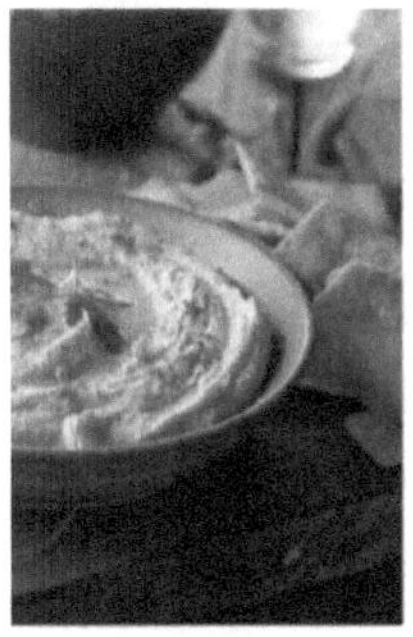

Lentil Hummus!

Ingredients

1 1/2 cup dry split red lentils, rinsed
2 tablespoon olive oil
2 tablespoons lemon juice
2 cloves garlic, minced
1 jalapeno pepper
1 yellow onion
½ teaspoon smoked paprika
dash of cayenne pepper
1 teaspoon of hot sauce
3 tablespoon tahini – sesame seed paste
1 teaspoon ground cumin
sea salt to taste
ground black pepper to taste
3 ½ cups vegetable broth

Preparation

Heat the oil in a large pot over medium heat. Add onion until translucent or softened. Add the garlic, cumin, and paprika and cook about 2 minutes. Stir in the water and lentils; bring to a boil. Reduce the heat to medium low, cover and simmer until lentils are soft, about 15 minutes.

Add the contents to food processor with the hot sauce, cayenne pepper, jalapeno pepper, tahini, salt and pepper and pulse until smooth. Taste and adjust spices according to your liking. Transfer mixture to serving container. Sprinkle paprika on top before serving. Serve with bread, carrots and celery sticks.

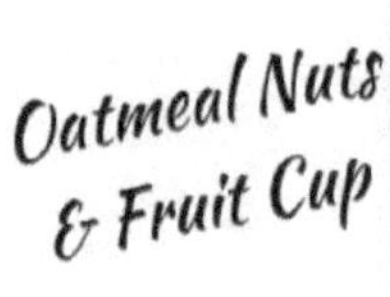

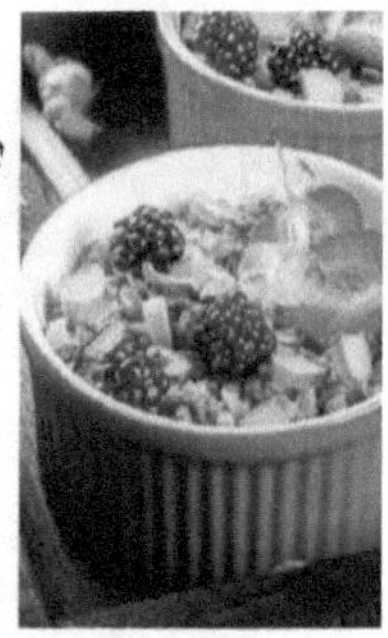

Ingredients

¾ cup rolled oats
1 ½ cup water
sea salt
¼ cup fresh berries (strawberries, blueberries, blackberries)
orange slice (optional)
kiwi slices (optional)

¼ teaspoon ground cinnamon
2 tablespoon dried fruit (raisins, dates, cranberries, etc)
2 tablespoons chopped nuts (pecans, walnuts, almonds, cashews)
sprinkle of Chia seeds
raw honey (optional)

Preparation

Combine the rolled oats and the water in a saucepan. Bring to a boil over high heat. Reduce to medium heat until the water is absorbed, about 5-7 minutes.

Stir in the cinnamon and salt Serve in a bowl or cup. Add the oats, then the berries, nuts, Chia seeds, and drizzle with the honey. Serve while hot.

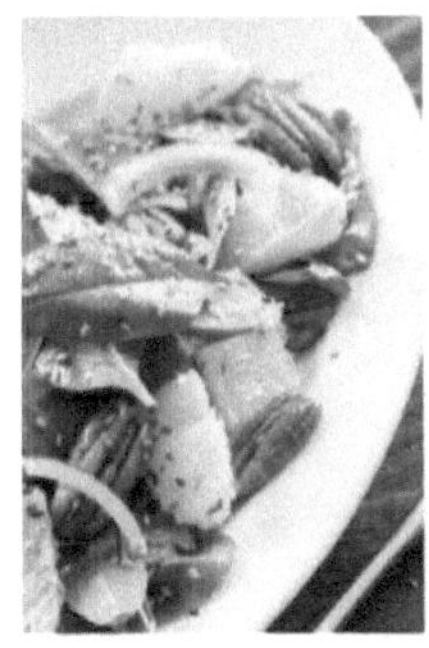

Spinach, Pecan & Orange Salad

Ingredients

4 cups fresh spinach
1 cup mandarin oranges
½ cup mushrooms

1 medium sweet onion, chopped
2 fresh boiled eggs. sliced
¼ cup walnuts (optional)
warm honey mustard dressing or cool cucumber dressing (recipe above)

Preparation

In a large bowl add the fresh spinach with the stems removed. Layer the other ingredients on top, mushrooms. onions and the oranges. Add the warm honey mustard dressing over the mixture and toss together. Upon serving add the boiled eggs on top.

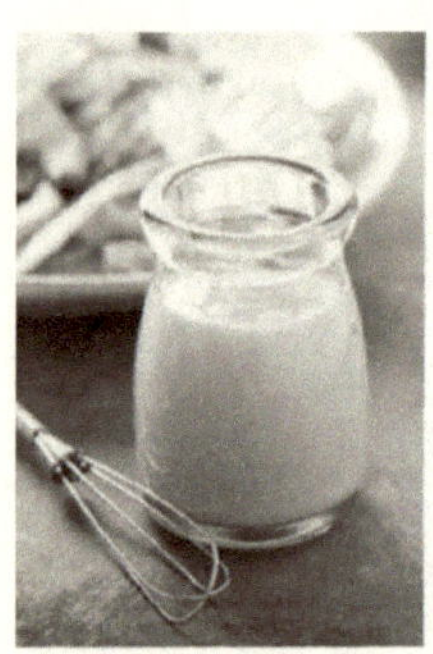

Ingredients

½ teaspoon Dijon mustard
3 tablespoons red wine vinegar
3 tablespoons sugar
Salt to taste
2 -3 Tablespoons bacon drippings

Preparation

In a heated pan add the bacon drippings and sugar, make sure it is mixed well. Add 3 tablespoon of the red wine vinegar and Dijon mustard. Make sure mixture is stirred and mixed well. Add salt to taste.

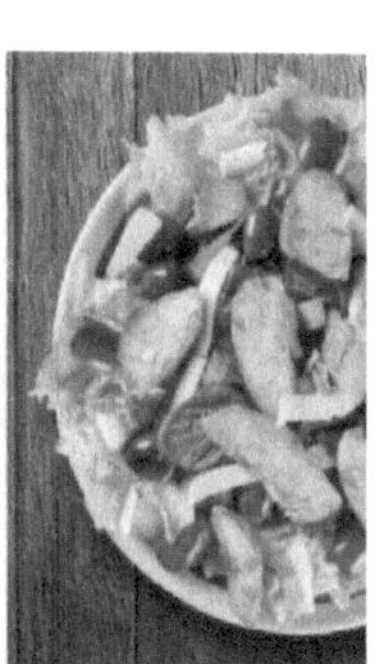

Ingredients

2 cups fresh spring salad mix
½ package of roasted herb chicken, shredded
1 cup chopped apple slices
¼ cups chopped sweet walnuts
¼ cup chopped red onion
½ cup balsamic dressing
1 tablespoon of olive oil
salt and fresh ground pepper to taste

Preparation

Preheat wok to medium heat. Add the olive oil. Add the chicken and cook until thoroughly cooked on both sides. Remove from heat and drain, if needed.

Toss the spring salad mix, apples, walnuts, red onions, salt, pepper, and dressing. Make sure everything is coated.

Add the ingredients to plate and add the chicken on top or you can add the chicken to the tossed ingredients.

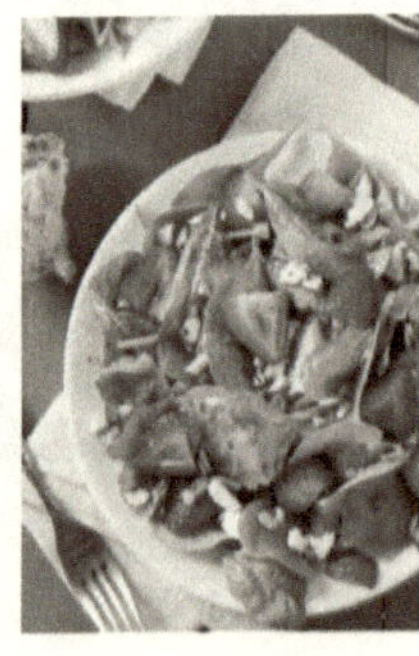

Strawberry Salad!

Ingredients

4 cups chopped romaine lettuce
3 cups fresh strawberries
1 cup red grapes
¼ cup sliced almonds
¼ cup red onion
avocado
may add feta cheese or bleu cheese
2 cups grilled chicken breast cooked
salt and fresh ground pepper to taste
½ cup poppy seed dressing (Marzetti)

Preparation

In a large bowl toss the romaine, strawberries, chicken, grapes, onion, cheese and almonds. Drizzle over the salad the poppy seed dressing.

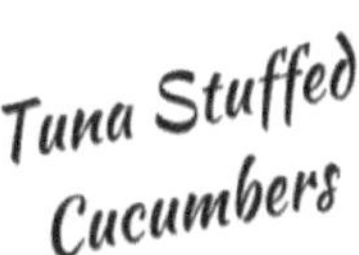

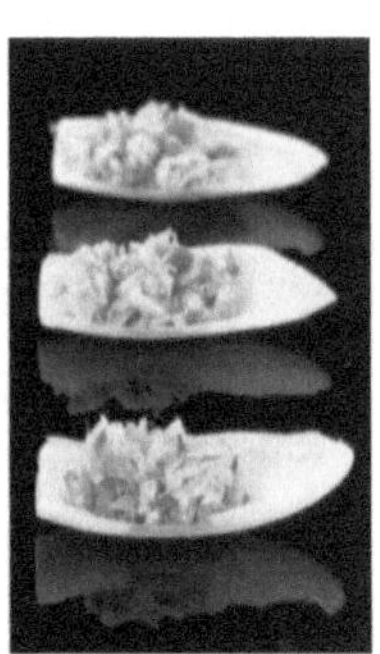

Ingredients

1 - 5 oz. can of tuna in water, drained and flaked
fresh parsley, chopped
diced onion
diced tomato
diced red bell pepper
olive oil
salt and fresh ground pepper
vinegar
3 cucumbers medium

Preparation

Drain the tuna and place in a large bowl. Add all ingredients to the bowl and seasoned to taste with olive oil, salt and pepper.

Clean cucumbers and cut in half lengthwise. You may remove skin from cucumber, remove and discard seeds. Cut a thin slice from the bottom of cucumber for them to sit flat. Spoon the tuna mixture into the cucumbers. Serve immediately.

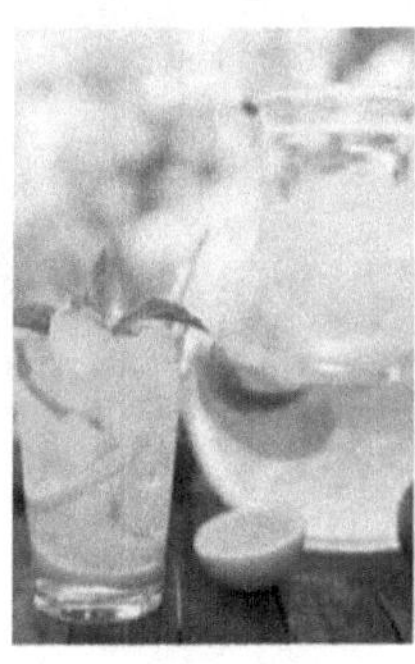

Lemon Cooler!

Ingredients

½ lemon, squeezed
8 ounces of water
4 ounces of ginger tea (I use ginger tea bags from my local organic store)

Add all ingredients in a glass to start your day. Drink every morning as a detoxification drink on an empty stomach. Best to drink room temperature. Can also drink lukewarm. This can be used as a liver detoxification. Take it for 3 days as a cleanse.

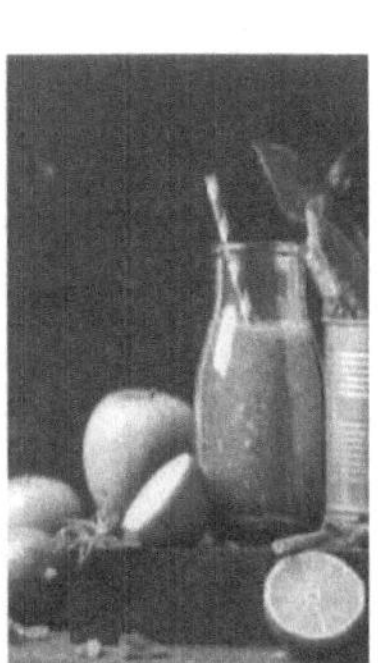

Ingredients

½ cup kiwi
1 green apple
1 ½ cup spinach
¼ cup cucumbers
juice of one orange
½ half banana
1 ½ unsweetened almond milk

Preparation

Chop and slice up the cucumbers, bananas, kiwi, apple, and the spinach.

Add all ingredients into blender and blend for several minutes until smooth in consistency. Pour in glass. Enjoy.

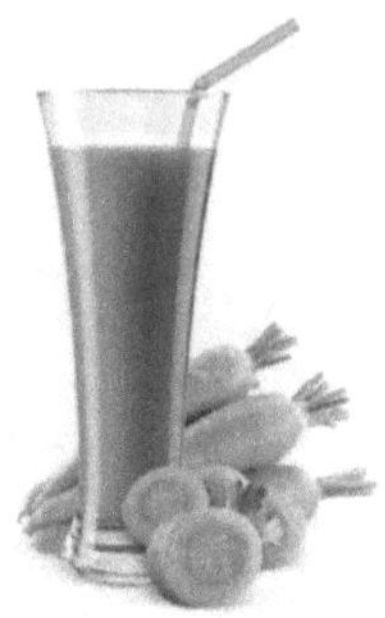

Carrot Juice

Ingredients

1 cup celery, diced
2 large carrots, peeled and sliced
1 medium apple, peeled and sliced
1 cup water

Preparation

Add all ingredients into blender and blend for several minutes until smooth in consistency. Pour in glass. Enjoy.

Juicy Juice!

Ingredients

1 stick celery, diced
1 medium apple, peeled and sliced
1/2 beetroot
2 carrots
1/2 cucumber
1 orange
lemon juice

Preparation

Add all ingredients into juicer. Pour in glass. Enjoy.

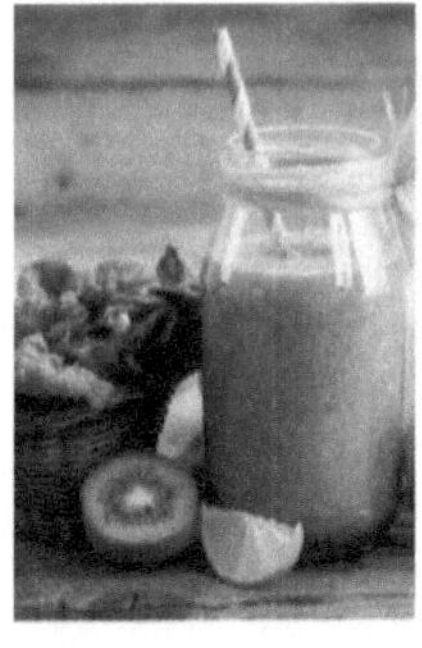

*Greens
Smoothie!*

Ingredients

2 sticks of celery
1 green apple
¼ pink grapefruit
1 pear
pinch of ginger, if not using fresh
pinch of turmeric, if not using fresh
mint leaves (optional)

Preparation

Cut up the celery, apple, and the pear. Finely chop the mint leaves.

Add apple, celery, and pear into juicer. Add ginger, turmeric. Add grapefruit. Pour in glass. Use the mint as garnish. Enjoy.

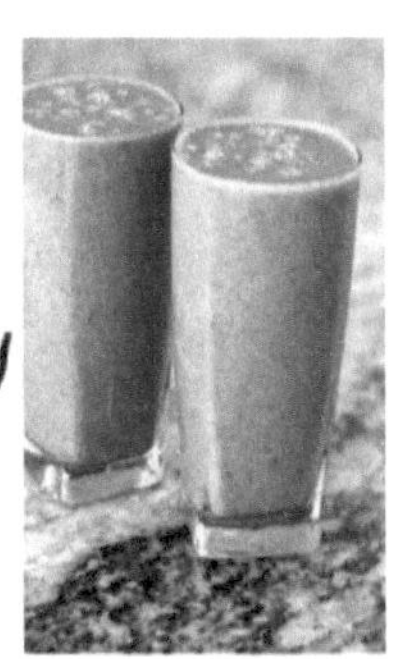

Submitted by: Vickie Marlin
Ingredients

1 cup almond milk
1 banana
1 cup kale leaves, de-stemmed
3 large strawberries

Add all to blender and blend until smooth. Enjoy.

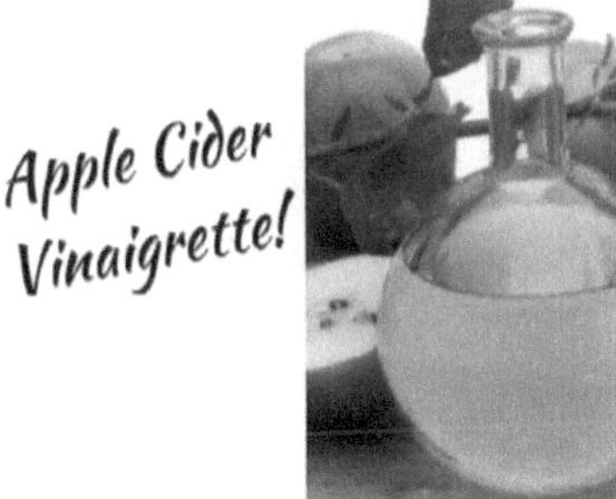

Ingredients

1 cup apple cider vinegar

¼ cup extra virgin olive oil
2 teaspoons crushed mustard seed
dash of sea salt
dash of fresh ground black pepper
Romano cheese

Mix all in a container and set aside to marinate and set for about 2 weeks. Make sure it is in airtight container or mason jar. This helps that all the content is mixed properly.

You may use some of the dressing but the flavor will be injected when the mixture has set for 2 weeks. It gets better over time.

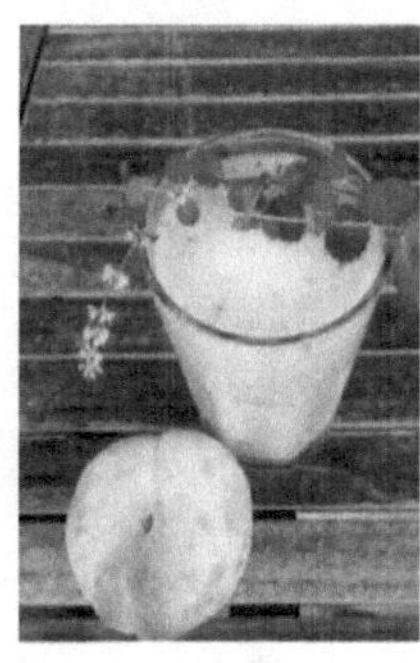

Strawberry, Peach, Banana Split Smoothie!

Ingredients

1/2 cup strawberries
1/2 cup mango, diced
½ banana, sliced

3 cherries to taste, pitted
1 6 oz. Greek yogurt plain
1/2 cup ice, to thicken

Preparation

Combine all ingredients in a blender and blend until smooth. Drink immediately.

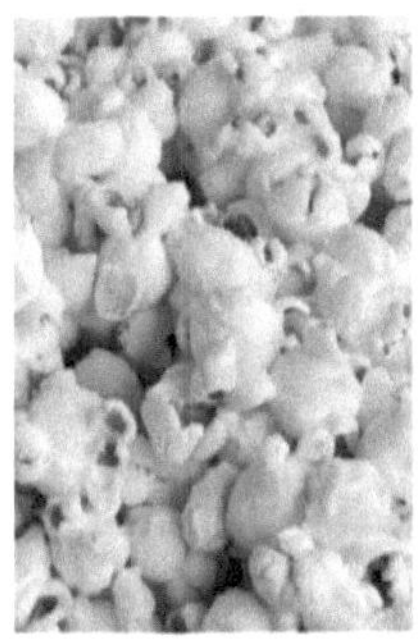

Skinny Popcorn, Coconut, Almonds, Granola, Chia Seeds Treat

Ingredients

1 bag 4.4 oz. Skinny Popcorn
1 bag 6 oz. Sliced Almonds
1 cup fresh coconut
2 Tablespoons Chia Seeds
1 Tablespoon Extra Virgin Olive Oil
½ cup Granola
½ cup Golden raisins
1 teaspoon Ground Cinnamon
Black Pepper to taste

Preparation
Combine all ingredients in a large bowl and toss together. Enjoy as a snack. May store in a zip lock bag for 1-2 days.

[a] Frequencies, http://isira.com/wordpress/wp-content/uploads/2011/06/YL-Essential-Oils-Frequency-LA.pdf

[b] Heavenly Frequencies, http://johntussey.com/

[c] Wholetones, https://wholetones.com/

[d] Essential Oils, http://isira.com/wordpress/wp-content/uploads/2011/06/YL-Essential-Oils-Frequency-LA.pdf

[e] Reference Guide to Essential Oils and Healing Oils of the Bible

ABOUT THE AUTHOR

Janet A. Cooksey is an author, speaker, life coach and an executive that loves to build up "Champions" no matter what sphere of influence you find yourself whether in ministry or business. She loves to see everyone healed, whole and walking in freedom. She is a healing and deliverance minister with signs, wonders and miracles following.

She is Co-Lead to the COH-IAM Ministry which is mandated: to assist the saints to become a bride fully prepared for Him -- glorious and radiant, beautiful and holy, without fault or flaw via love encounters and to set the captives free by sharing information that will equip them to learn to have the confidence to boldly enter into His Courts for themselves and seek His face. This is His heart cry to us -- that all engage with Him directly.

Janet is available for speaking engagements upon request. She can be reached at RaphaHeartMinistries@gmail.com for information regarding resources, itinerary, or to schedule a ministry appointment.

For business appointments contact Janet at SavvyIntelSolutions@gmail.com for life coaching for career and business development support and resources.
Janet has one wonderful son and resides in Baltimore-Washington Metropolitan Region.